MEDICAL PARENTING

HOW TO NAVIGATE HEALTH, WELLNESS & THE MEDICAL SYSTEM WITH YOUR CHILD

Jacqueline Jones, MD

M·J

NEW YORK

LONDON • NASHVILLE • MELBOURNE • VANCOUVER

MEDICAL PARENTING

How to Navigate Health, Wellness & the Medical System with Your Child

Published in New York, New York, by Morgan James Publishing. Morgan James is a trademark of Morgan James, LLC. www.MorganJamesPublishing.com

The information provided in this book represents the opinions of the author and is designed to provide helpful information on the subjects discussed. This book is not meant to be used, nor should it be used, to diagnose or treat any medical condition. For diagnosis or treatment of any medical problem, consult a physician. The author is not responsible for any specific legal, health, or allergy needs that may require medical supervision or consultation with an attorney, and is not liable for any damages or negative consequences from any treatment, action, application or preparation, to any person reading or following the information in this book.

All information is provided "as is" and "as available" without warranties of any kind, expressed or implied, including accuracy, timeliness, and completeness. In no instance should a user attempt to diagnose a medical condition or determine appropriate treatment based on the information contained in this book. All forms and figures contained in this book are examples and should not be used for legal or medical purposes. Figures, forms and references are provided for informational purposes only and do not constitute endorsement of any websites or other sources. Readers should be aware that the websites listed in this book may change. To protect the privacy of certain individuals, the names and identifying details have been changed.

ISBN 9781642794502 paperback
ISBN 9781642794519 eBook
Library of Congress Control Number: 2019900582

Cover and Interior Design by:
Mido Emad, Susan Veach

Edited by:
Rebecca Daigle, Cecilia Levine

Dedication

To my husband John - your love and support have been the bedrock of my life for 35 years.

To my children, who have taught me unconditional love, I am so very proud of the men you have become.

To the families who have allowed me to become a part of your lives - I have been honored to share the path to health with you and your children.

"No one is ever quite ready;
everyone is always caught off guard.
Parenthood chooses you.
And you open your eyes,
look at what you've got, say "Oh, my gosh,"
and recognize that of all the balls there ever were,
this is the one you should not drop.
It is not a question of choice."

Marisa de los Santos,
author of *Love Walked In*

Contents

Foreword

So you need parenting advice in the information age? What could be easier! Medical question about your 5-month-old, energetic bundle of joy who seems to have eaten a generous piece of your 3-day-old pepperoni pizza while you were momentarily distracted by a preview on Netflix? Not to worry. You take out your smartphone and consult, as doctors in training say, "Dr. Google." And presto, there is the answer! Well, a few answers. Start to scroll, and you find there are way too many answers. To take a short break from your medical search, you navigate over to Facebook and now see ads for super-absorbent diapers guaranteed not to leak. Sort of interesting, but at the moment, probably not at the top of your to-do list. At least, you hope not. It may be time to update your status.

When it comes to medical care, being surrounded by constant information and advice has not made parenting easier. Along with the fast-paced changes that have come with the information age, are the ever more complex medical systems that provide our health care. Navigating the medical system as a parent can be challenging, frustrating, and sometimes quite frightening. Your goal is to give your child the best medical care possible. Where to start? What steps to take? How to do this?

This is where Dr. Jacqueline Jones' remarkable new book, *Medical Parenting: How to Navigate Health, Wellness and the Medical System with Your Child* comes in. As a parent and physician, Dr. Jones brings a great combination of knowledge, experience, compassion, and personal perspective to provide parents a much-needed roadmap of today's medical system. From how best to choose a doctor, to emergencies, all the way from early childhood through the teenage years, Dr. Jones gives clear, sound advice. Not only will you enjoy reading this book, you will also gain confidence as a parent and help ensure that your child stays well and gets the best health care possible.

Take it from a father of four who also happens to be a physician: Read this book and keep it by your bed next to your smartphone. When you need sound guidance, I know which device you'll reach for. Sorry, Dr. Google—Dr. Jones is on call tonight.

Peter C. Adamson, MD

Professor of Pediatrics & Pharmacology

Perelman School of Medicine, University of Pennsylvania

Children's Hospital of Philadelphia

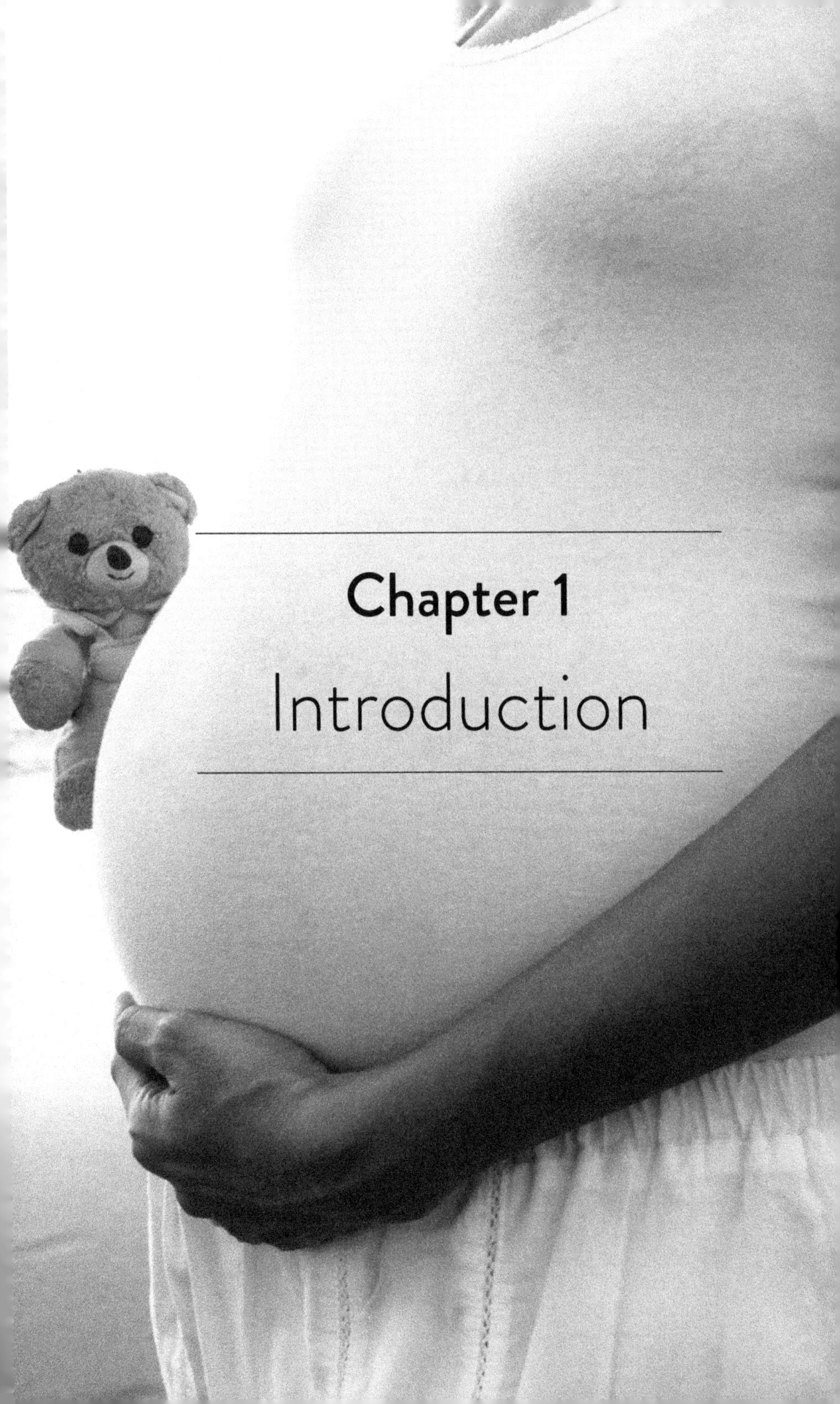

Chapter 1
Introduction

This love was different.
It was intense.
It was a love that
I have never known before.

I stood in the dim light of the radiology department's reading room at the prestigious New York City Hospital, looking at my newborn son's CT scan of his brain. It was the same hospital where I worked, but that day, my pink robe and fluffy slippers were in vivid contrast to the stark white of the lab coat, draped over my dear friend and radiologist, now caring for my son.

"Don't worry, Jackie. It's just the front part of his brain that's damaged," she told me. "He probably doesn't need that anyway."

My colleagues at the hospital knew me as congenial, friendly, and easy to work with. That day, with my son as a patient, I was anything but.

"You have got to be fu—king kidding me!" I shrieked. "Get the neurologist up here now. I want this fixed."

The emotions that ran through me in those moments were primal. I would protect this child at any cost and I would claw through anyone who stood in my way. I had delayed having children until I finished my rigorous surgical residency. Being awake for 36 hours at a time and stumbling home to sleep for 10 hours, only to start again the next morning, was too grueling on my body to even think about becoming pregnant.

My husband, who was five years my senior, was anxious to start a family, and during my final year of training, I agreed. As usual, I had everything planned to the minute.

I would get pregnant in November, deliver in July and have time to recover before starting my job in September. It was the first of many lessons I would learn as a mother: my child would do things on his schedule—not mine.

It took several months for me to conceive, and when my son was born, I was working 12-hour days, 6 days a week and was reluctant to take any time off to prepare myself for his arrival. My labor and delivery were long and difficult.

Fear gripped me as they lead my husband out of the delivery room, my obstetrician voicing concern over my condition.

"Jackie," he said, leaning over me, "the baby is too far down for a C-section, but he is stuck in your small pelvis. I'm going to use the forceps."

Agonizing minutes passed until I heard a cry that I shall remember for as long as I live. Shrill and piercing, it was music to my ears. The obstetrician tended to me as I held my baby in my arms, still unable to fathom the love that I felt for him.

I have felt love before—for my husband, my parents, and even my cats. But this love was different. It was intense. It was a love that I have never known before.

My baby was seen by the neurologist and remained hospitalized for several days, but he finally arrived home bundled in my arms and in my heart.

That same love for my two children has matured over the past two decades, and deepened in a way that is still difficult for me to fathom.

Being a mother, however, has also made me a more compassionate physician, as I better understand the depth of emotions and fear that is often elicited for parents and caretakers entering the medical system with their children.

With this book, I hope to impart my experience as a mother and a physician to help you better navigate the medical system you must interact with as a loving and responsible parent.

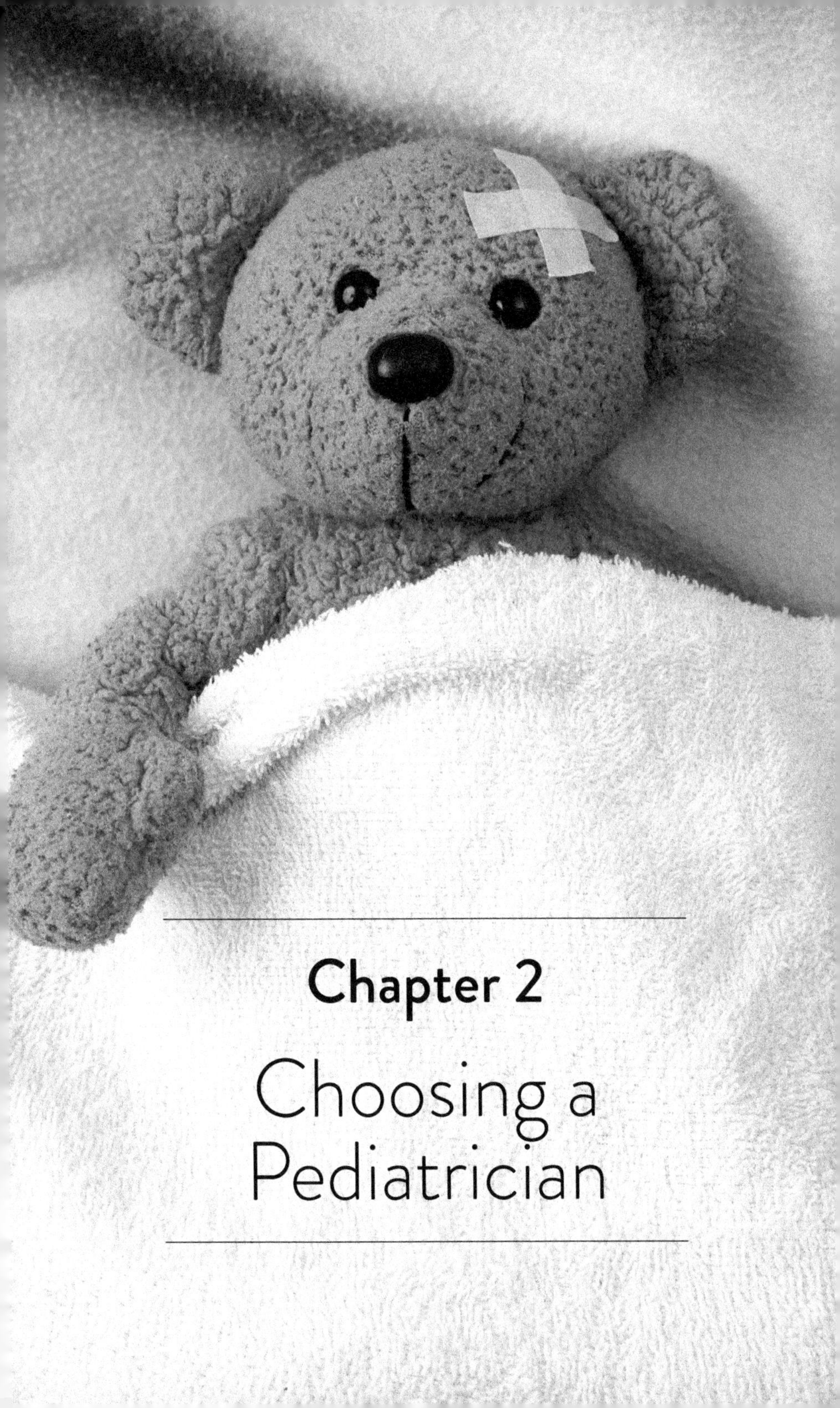

Chapter 2

Choosing a Pediatrician

I had done the best I could
to support this mother.

The marriage you enter into with your pediatrician can last for more than 21 years, so buyer beware: it is important to spend time deciding what type of person you are, and what type of support and availability you will need.

The following story may have played out much differently, had the patient's parents spent more time finding a pediatrician better suited to their situation.

I reached down and laid my hand on the shoulder of the sobbing mother who sat in my exam chair, her small child nestled in her arms.

"It is going to be okay, we'll figure this out together," I reassured her. Her newborn child was having problems breastfeeding and I could feel the anxiety and sense of failure radiating from her hunched shoulders.

She had driven more than two hours from her home in Connecticut to see me, searching for answers and a solution to the escalating daily battles between her and her infant. I had found a tongue-tie in this perfectly formed baby boy, something relatively common in newborns. That paired with his mother's inexperience with breastfeeding had turned what should have been an enjoyable bonding experience for a mother and child into a frustrating and painful ordeal for them both.

The solution involved a five-minute procedure to snip

the excess tissue anchoring the tongue. As I described the procedure, the mother dissolved into tears.

"I can't do it," she sobbed. "I'm not strong enough. There must be another way."

I gently suggested calling her husband for support, but he was at work and unavailable. Recognizing this fact seemed to make her even more upset. Things were not looking good.And so, I called her pediatrician—a medical practice I was not familiar with—and was greeted with the proverbial phone tree. It rang and rang for minutes until a real human finally greeted me.

"May I speak to the doctor about one of his patients in need of some guidance?" I asked.

The secretary on the other end was curt and brisk: "One minute," she snapped.

It was not one minute—it was six and a half. But I practiced deep breathing as the young mother's sobs resonated in the otherwise quiet exam room.

"Don't worry," I cooed as I waited on the phone. I tried to exude calm and patience, even though it was truly not what I was feeling at that moment. "Yes," a male voice boomed in the phone. Finally!

I explained the burden this poor mother was carrying, feeling inadequate and alone in her first few days of motherhood. I discussed my recommendations and asked if she might reach out to him later that day so he could discuss her options.

"Sorry, I'm really busy. Just tell her to go ahead with the procedure," the doctor barked into the phone before hanging up. Click.

Obviously, that was not what this mother needed. She needed guidance, support, and someone she trusted to help her make the decision she faced. No matter how friendly and supportive I might try to be, I was a stranger, unable to impartially advise on the path to follow.

It is crucial when choosing a pediatrician to recognize if you are the type of parent who needs frequent support and reinforcement as you parent your child, or if you feel confident about your parenting skills and need only occasional advice. Choose a practice that suits your needs in order to alievate frustration for both you and your pediatrician.

I did the best that I could, but I was not her doctor. I was not who that mother needed.

"Let's put this off for few days," I said. "Make an appointment to see your pediatrician and discuss this more fully. It's not a life-threatening situation. I don't want to rush you."

The sobbing intensified and now the baby, perhaps sensing his mother's despair, began to wail. I opened the door and beckoned my most patient assistant.

"Alison will take you to my office to call your mom or husband to come get you," I told the mother, still crying in the room. "No rush, please stay with us as long as you need to."

It was a failure for us all. I had done the best I could to support this mother. The baby did not receive the care I felt would be beneficial in helping him to adequately breastfeed, and this mother obviously was distraught. Then there was me, feeling frustrated and annoyed that I could not make a difference for this child and his mother.

Had her pediatrician or a member of his staff been more available for this mother, I believe she would have felt more supported and able to make an informed decision that would have helped both her and her child.

Choosing a pediatrician/primary caregiver is one of the most important decisions you will make as you enter the medical system. A recommendation from your obstetrician is an excellent place to start.

If you had a good working relationship with your obstetrician over the course of your pregnancy, it is likely that they will refer you to a pediatrician or family practitioner with a similar philosophy and style of practice. Ask your obstetrician why they recommend a certain practice and the length of time they have worked with that practice.Recommendations from family and friends are important resources; however, who your mother-in-law feels is the best pediatrician in the area may not fit your lifestyle or expectations for care. Instead, consider asking friends and family members with similar views to yours who they would recommend.

There is no substitute for doing your homework and researching practitioners yourself.

Some things to consider when choosing a practitioner:

- **Your personality.** It is vital that you and your partner are brutally honest with each other about your needs and expectations.

- **Where you live.** Your geographic location can be limiting. If you live in a rural area with one large pediatric practice, your decision is likely made for you. If you live in an urban area, there may be 50 or more pediatric practices close by to choose from.

Here are a few of the questions you should ask yourself to determine which practice is right for you.

- Are you comfortable developing a casual relationship with many different practitioners in the practice, or do you prefer seeing your pediatrician for the majority of your visits?
- Do you need a pediatrician with years of experience, or would you like a younger person who might be at a similar stage in life as you and your partner?
- Are you opposed to seeing physician extenders, such as physician's assistants or nurse practitioners?
- Does the pediatrician participate with your insurance? In the first three months of life, you will need to see your pediatrician at least three times. It is likely you may need to go more frequently. Have your insurance card in hand when you call the office or check the website. Large insurance companies have many different plans and you will need to know exactly which plan you have to assure coverage. Make sure that you have alerted your insurance company that you will be adding your child to your policy. In the event you have chosen a pediatrician who does not accept your insurance, call

the office and get a fee schedule so there are no surprises when you are seen in the office on a Saturday or as an emergency. Ask for the fees for routine and emergency office visits, vaccinations, blood tests, and hearing and vision screening.

- Is the phone answered in the doctor's office, or triaged to a phone bank and then referred to the doctor's practice? Will it annoy you to not know any of the telephone support staff you will interact with?
- How will emergencies be handled if you have one during the night or weekend? If you call, will you speak to a physician—or a nursing service that screens all calls? Are there office hours on the weekend and how will those hours be staffed? If the doctor is away from the office, will you need to be seen in a different location or will an on-call doctor see you at the physician's office?
- Is the physician open to the use of alternative medications if that is an area of medicine you feel is important to your child's health? Does the physician's office work with any pharmacies or practitioners to ensure you are only giving the highest quality supplements to your child?
- If you are a working parent and cannot attend every appointment, how does the office convey information to you about your child's visit (i.e., a written report, verbal communication)? Can you join the visit via Skype?
- If you have concerns about vaccinations, is the physi-

cian open to considering options for nonessential vaccinations?

- What is the physician's view on breastfeeding? If you are unable (or unwilling) to breastfeed, will the pediatrician be able to work with you? As you work through your decision to breastfeed or bottle-feed, allow your pediatrician to work with you. Studies have shown that breastfeeding is the best source of nutrition for your newborn child; however, there are excellent formulas available that can be used in the place of breastfeeding or to supplement your child's feeding.[1] Ultimately, the choice on how to feed your child is yours, and a good pediatrician should respect that.

- Studies have shown there is a slight increase in infection in uncircumcised men but this risk is low.[2] Your pediatrician should be open to discussing these risks and open to your decision. If you do not want to circumcise your son, will the pediatrician support that?

- Can routine blood work be done in the physician's office, or do you need to go to a commercial lab? If blood work is done in the office, will a doctor or nurse be drawing the blood?

- As your child ages, are there options for switching pediatricians within the practice? Your teenager may feel more comfortable discussing questions about sex with a physician of the same gender, though any skilled pediatrician can help steer your child through this process.

- Would you prefer using a primary care physician instead of a pediatrician? A primary care physician has the advantage of following your child into adulthood. They can also provide comprehensive family care by caring for all members of the family.

Social media: Social Media and the internet can have a significant impact on the process of choosing a physician. There are multiple sites available to research your options.

Blogging sites: Many parenting sites are available for reference. Start by searching for parenting sites in your neighborhood. They will be the best sites for up-to-date information about pediatricians close to your home. Assure that the site has recommendations from multiple sources. Try to remove as much bias as possible from the process by assuring that multiple voices give input into a particular practice.

Yelp: Cross-check the names you have found on national sites such as Yelp. Realize that people who have had negative experiences may be more likely to post than the hundreds who have had good experiences. These sites may help give you an idea of the good points and bad points a practice may have. I would be much more likely to go to a practice where the negative comments surround a wait for an excellent practitioner as compared to someone with a poor bedside manner, or worse—an incompetent physician.

American Academy of Pediatrics (AAP): The AAP maintains a list of its members. Their website is a wonderful starting point to researching physicians' qualifications and credentials. You may want to consider AAP members as this suggests they will be knowledgeable and have access to this national organization's recommendations and standards of care.

Local hospitals: You have already gone to the trouble of researching local hospitals and choosing an obstetrician associated with a hospital where you feel comfortable receiving your care. Contact your hospital's physician referral service to receive a list of names of physicians associated with that hospital. While the hospital you have chosen may have extensive obstetrical services, be sure to assess that the pediatrics department meets your standards and expectations. This can be done by doing a search of the number of pediatric admissions the hospital has per year. Research if the hospital has a pediatrician available in the emergency room on nights and weekends. If there is a problem with your child after delivery, who will care for them? Most hospitals now employ hospitalists to care for inpatients. Does your hospital employ pediatric hospitalists and will your pediatrician be allowed to be involved with the care of your newborn?

State medical societies: Many state medical societies have data banks of physicians who are members of its medical society. You can obtain information about their address, hospital affiliations, certifications by the American Board of Medical Specialties, and their insurance company participation.

The Association of Primary Care Physicians: If your decision is to choose a primary care physician instead of a pediatrician, research the practice thoroughly. Many primary care physicians provide excellent pediatric care and have the advantage of caring for your entire family during all stages of your family's life. The Association of Primary Care Medicine can be a resource in finding a physician in your area who has a vibrant pediatric component to their practice. Contact your local hospital to help determine what practices are affiliated with your local hospital.

Once you have completed your research, you may consider meeting your potential caregiver in person.

Know yourself: Is establishing a connection with a pediatrician important to you prior to your child's birth, or are you comfortable with developing that connection after his or her delivery? Many pediatric practices will have monthly meet-and-greet sessions where you can meet the physicians and nurse practitioners in a practice. This is a group session where other prospective parents will have the opportunity to have their questions answered as well.

Group sessions can be excellent opportunities to have many questions answered, even some that you did not think to ask. If you have special needs or are put off by asking your questions in a group setting, inquire about the availability of a one-on-one session. Most practitioners will charge for this time and it will not be covered by insurance, so setting the fee up front as well as the amount of time the practitioner will spend with you is important.

These are some of the factors that should go into your decision to choose a practice.

Location: During the first few months of your child's life, you will visit your child's pediatric practice many times. Consider which location is most convenient for you. If you do not drive and do not have access to quality public transportation, the practice should be close by. If you drive, is there parking nearby that is accessible and affordable? Check the satellite map of the practice and see what access there is to the office. If there is a flight of stairs and no elevator, and you have twins with a stroller, that might not be the best choice for you. Is there handicap access if you or child requires special access?

Size of the practice: There are advantages and disadvantages to both large and small practices. In a smaller practice, you have the opportunity to see the same physician for the majority of your visits. This will hopefully promote a deeper and more personal relationship with your health-care provider, with the increased opportunity for you to interact with each other.

The disadvantage of a small practice is that when your

pediatrician is unavailable, you will need to see another physician and may be required to visit another practice location to receive care from the covering physician. Emergency calls will also be handled by a call group of physicians who you may not have had the opportunity to meet.

A large practice has advantages of its own. Primarily, it allows you the ability to always be seen during regular office hours. Night and weekend calls will usually be covered by the practice, so there is a higher chance of your knowing the physician who answers your emergency call. If your child needs to be seen for an emergency, his or her primary pediatrician may not see them—but rest assured that their primary physician will have ready access to the care your child received in the practice.

A large practice also affords you the ability to receive opinions from other physicians on issues of concern. Larger practices, in most instances, have a diversity of physicians with different ages and personalities, although their practice philosophies will be similar.

Concierge practices: In a concierge medical practice, you are hiring a private physician or small practice. Concierge practices charge a membership fee that can be up to several thousand dollars per year.

Memberships may include all office visits, or the doctor may charge per visit or submit your visits to your insurance company for reimbursement.

In most concierge practices, your membership fee allows

you 24/7 access to the physician, same-day appointments, minimal wait time upon arrival, and coordination of care with your child's specialist if needed. Most concierge practices provide weekend appointments and home visits though there might be an additional charge for these services. If you have the resources and desire for this type of care, there are increasing options for this level of service for your child.

Making the right decision:

Choosing your child's primary care provider:

Your face-to-face meeting with your child's potential primary care provider is your opportunity to ask the questions that will help you feel comfortable choosing a doctor and practice. It is imperative that both you and your spouse/partner attend these sessions. This must be a family decision as each of you will pick up on different information provided by the practice and can compare and contrast your opinions. Talk freely with your partner and make this important decision together. If you are having real trouble choosing between two different practices, go back to each and spend an hour in the waiting room chatting with other parents, observing the flow of the practice and how the front desk and support staff interacts with their patients. If you attended a group face-to-face session and would like more personal time with a potential primary care provider, you can call the office to inquire about booking a private session with the physician. Expect to be charged for this time.

Anxiety around your child's health during the first several weeks, months, and years is part of being a parent.

Learning how to channel that anxiety into positive action is an important step in supporting yourself and your child. The more information you can gather prior to those first tumultuous weeks after your delivery will help you deal with whatever life has in store for you and your child.

Chapter 3

Primary Care Physician

Building a rapport with your primary care physician

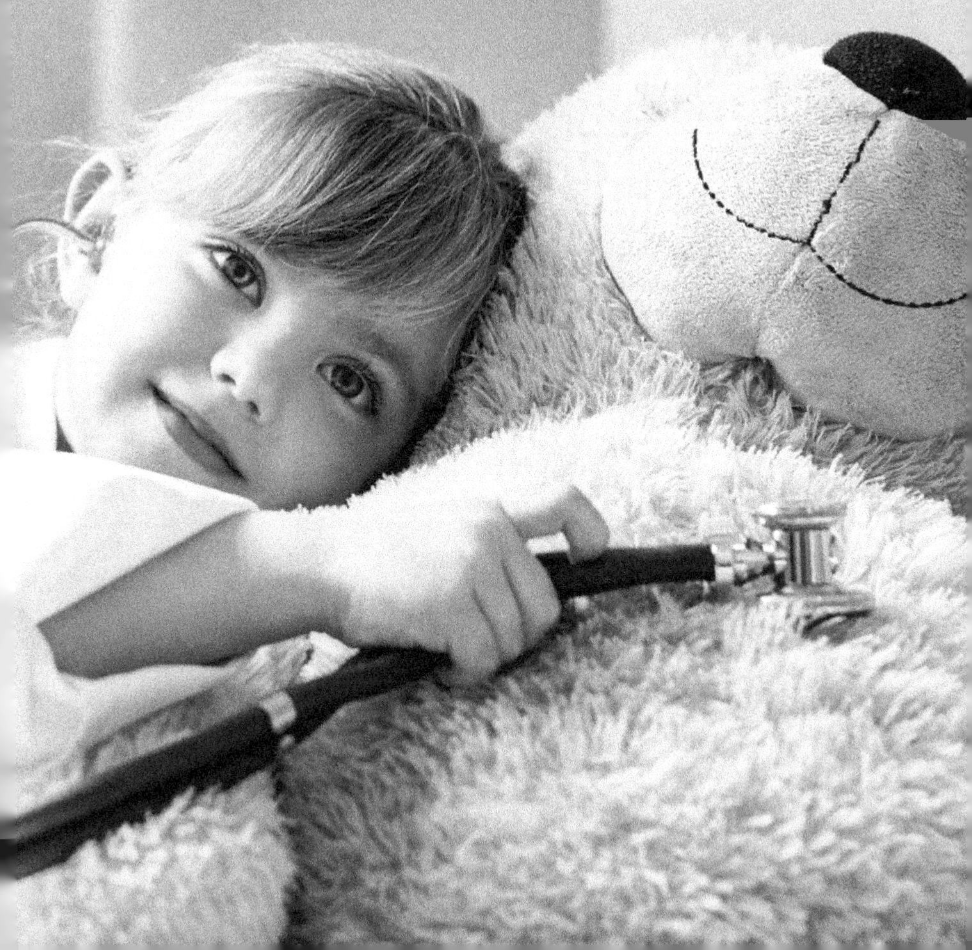

The relationship you form with your pediatrician is vital to your child's health.

Warm, golden light flooded through the hospital windows as I sat next to my newborn's incubator. But inside, darkness penetrated every fiber of my being.

The pale blue, late-March sky was reflecting in the monitor that was mounted above my boy, causing me to squint every time I went to check his vital signs, which occured every few minutes.

I felt out of control and at a loss. I did not know how to help my fragile child. My husband slept slumped in the chair beside me, his rhythmic breathing and warmth doing nothing to cut through the chill that emanated from deep inside me.

I had completed four years of medical school, six years of residency and one year of fellowship taking care of babies just like this—why couldn't I fix my own? Why did I have to be one of those mothers I had breezed in to gaze upon for the past decade?

My hair was pulled into a ponytail, my face was devoid of makeup, and my clothes were rumpled and creased from hours perched on the stiff chairs of the large neonatal intensive care unit. I was worn and frazzled. Looking at my reflection in the mirror of the small bathroom next to my child's room, I did not recognize the dark, blank stare that greeted me. I could see the looks that the nurses—who I had worked with over the past year—gave me as they tended to my child.

"Dr. Jones, why don't you go home and get some rest?" they suggested. "At least go downstairs and get something to eat."

Surely if I left his side, something bad would happen. As long as I was there, certainly I could influence fate, prevent any misfortune that lurked in the vast unknown from reaching him.

It had been three days and I knew in my heart that I was in a bad place. I knew rationally as an intelligent human being and physician that my presence would have no meaningful effect on the outcome, but as a mother—and a mother in crisis—these rational thoughts could not penetrate the terror and darkness that gripped me.My husband's eyes slowly opened and he reached for my hand. He pulled me up and led me to the couch in the waiting room.

"At least lie down for a few hours," he said. "I'll go home to sleep and be back later."

He watched as I lay down with the starchy crispness of a hospital blanket, wrapped over my head and body. I turned into the cool, plastic of the couch and allowed the exhaustion to overtake me.

"Jackie, Jackie, open your eyes," my friend and my child's pediatrician, said to me, perched on the corner of the couch, her hand resting on my shoulder. "I'm here."

The room was still and dark as the hospital settled into the quiet of its late-night pace.

The pediatrician I had chosen was not much older than I was, and had only been in practice for a handful of years. We had worked together on several difficult cases and I loved her commitment to patients and families, as well as her ability to connect on a personal level with both the families and staff.

"The nurses called me, Jackie," she said. "They are worried about you. They tell me you haven't left the unit in three days and you're not eating."

I stared blankly at her face and stammered something about being fine. She looked deep into my eyes, and I knew I wasn't fooling anyone.

"I've made you an appointment to see someone in the morning," she said. "You must go. If you need me to walk you over there, just call."

She pressed a piece of paper into my hand and my fingers slowly closed around it.

"Jackie, I'm watching your son closely and I promise you, we will do everything we can to get both of you through this."She rose and looked down as I struggled into a more dignified position.

"Just rest, he's fine," she said. "Call me anytime you need me. I'm here."

She turned and walked slowly out of the room and finally, after many days of holding back, I allowed the tears that had been so close to the surface to fall.

The relationship you form with your pediatrician is vital to your child's health. Non-verbal, immobile, and dependent on you for their survival, your child has no way to advocate for themselves. Your pediatrician relies on you to serve as the interpreter.

Remember your primary care provider is there to care for your child and help you to become an effective and supportive parent.

Making your first appointment: Your first interaction with your pediatrician or family physician will likely be at your first appointment. This is a critical time to set the tone for future interactions with the office. Introduce yourself as a new parent and be patient during the registration process. Many practices allow you to register online and this may serve as a handy tool, but do not underestimate the importance of a personal connection.

The examination: Your first appointment has arrived and you have a host of questions for the physician. Recognize that they also have a great deal of information that they would like to pass on to you—so be sensitive of their time. Do your homework, think through the important questions and write them down before you enter the exam room with your child.

If you have not interviewed your pediatrician during your prenatal stage, your first several visits should focus on dialogue that will help you and your pediatrician better understand each other. Asking what medical school and residency they attended and if they have ever been sued seems a waste of both your time and theirs. You have committed to this relationship. Concentrating on helping it to mature and develop will be the most useful for all.

Be present in the moment as your pediatrician interacts with you and your child. Turn off your cell phone and avoid checking your email while medical staff is in the room. There is nothing in your email that can't wait 20 minutes—and if you must answer the phone, apologize, step outside and make it quick.

As you develop this relationship, try to have both parents attend well-child visits. Acquainting yourself with your pediatrician during routine visits will make working together in the event of a crisis much easier. If work keeps you from attending appointments, and you want to be part of the interaction, discuss the possibility of Skype, FaceTime or phone calls during your child's visit with your health-care provider.

An extended family is an important part of many cultures. Pediatric health-care providers are sensitive to your need of having support as you go through the process of raising your child. However, your pediatric visit is not the best place to have that support out in full force.

Limit your visit to one additional person for support. I have walked into my exam room to find a small infant with two parents, four grandparents and a nanny. Fielding questions from multiple adults makes it more difficult for physicians to concentrate on the needs of the most important people, outside your child, in the room: the parents.

At some point during the visit, your pediatrician will examine your child. This can be stressful for new parents, as we work so hard to protect our newborns from anything that might upset them. Do not let your fears cloud the decision to allow your pediatrician to fully examine your child. Limiting which procedures are done to and for your child during an office visit should be thoroughly discussed if you have real concerns. Rest assured that your health-care provider has extensive experience in handling children, and will be gentle and careful when interacting with your child. Your child may cry during these examinations but will recover, as will you, just more slowly.

A dialogue between you and your child's health-care provider is vitally important, as they give you guidance and advice. If you feel that you will be distracted, bring your spouse, significant other, extended family member, or friend to take notes for you. You have your pediatrician's undivided attention during this time. Try to take every opportunity to give them yours as they give you advice and recommendations.

If medication is prescribed, it is important to ask your provider exactly what the medication is treating and if there are any side effects. Confirm any allergies your child may have to medications with your physician, and make sure that your physician is made aware of any allergies that you already know of. If you are hesitant to use medications or want to know more about the risks and benefits, discuss these concerns with your child's physician.

Phone contact: Your pediatrician's office is there to provide guidance and support during your journey with your child. Phone calls are a crucial part of that support. The practice of medicine is evolving, and the age of the small solo practice is fading. More and more practices will employ several health-care providers and physician extenders, such as nurse practitioners, physician's assistants, nurses, and medical assistants to assist them in your child's care.

When you call during the day, it is unlikely that you will have the opportunity to speak directly to your pediatrician—you would not want your appointment interrupted with someone else's routine calls. A physician extender will likely answer that call.

How do you interact with these health-care providers? You have every right to know with whom you are speaking, and their credentials. Give that individual as much medical information about your child as you can, such as allergies to foods or medication, when the symptoms started, and how severe they are. Writing a timeline before getting on the phone may help organize your thoughts as you voice your concerns.

Listen carefully to the advice provided and take notes so that your can refer to them later if you have any questions about the appropriate course of action. Be open to the fact that the staff has dealt with the vast majority of issues that you are calling about. However, if your child is truly experiencing an emergency, such as difficulty breathing, significant bleeding, or another life-threatening emergency, do insist on speaking with a physician immediately—or call 9-1-1.

If you feel uncomfortable with the information you are receiving and your call is not of an emergent nature, asking to have a physician call you back at the end of the day is appropriate. If you are the type of parent who prefers speaking only to a physician, choose your practice carefully. You might opt for a small practice or a concierge practice.

You chose your pediatric practice because you want only the best for your child, and every physician wants to provide that. No matter how good your pediatrician may be, there are some things that cannot be diagnosed over the phone, and insisting on medical treatment over the phone undermines that high level of care you are seeking. If you are advised to do so, make the trip to the office and let your pediatrician do what they do best: care for you and your child on a personal level.

The phone is an excellent way to follow up on tests that were taken during your visit. At the time of your visit, inquire how long it will take to get results and then place an alert in your phone to follow up on those results. It is rare for abnormal results to be missed, but a phone call from you will assure that you have the opportunity to review those results and hear a course of action to address any abnormalities.

Chapter 4

Interacting with Ancillary Care Staff

How to get the secretary to schedule an appointment

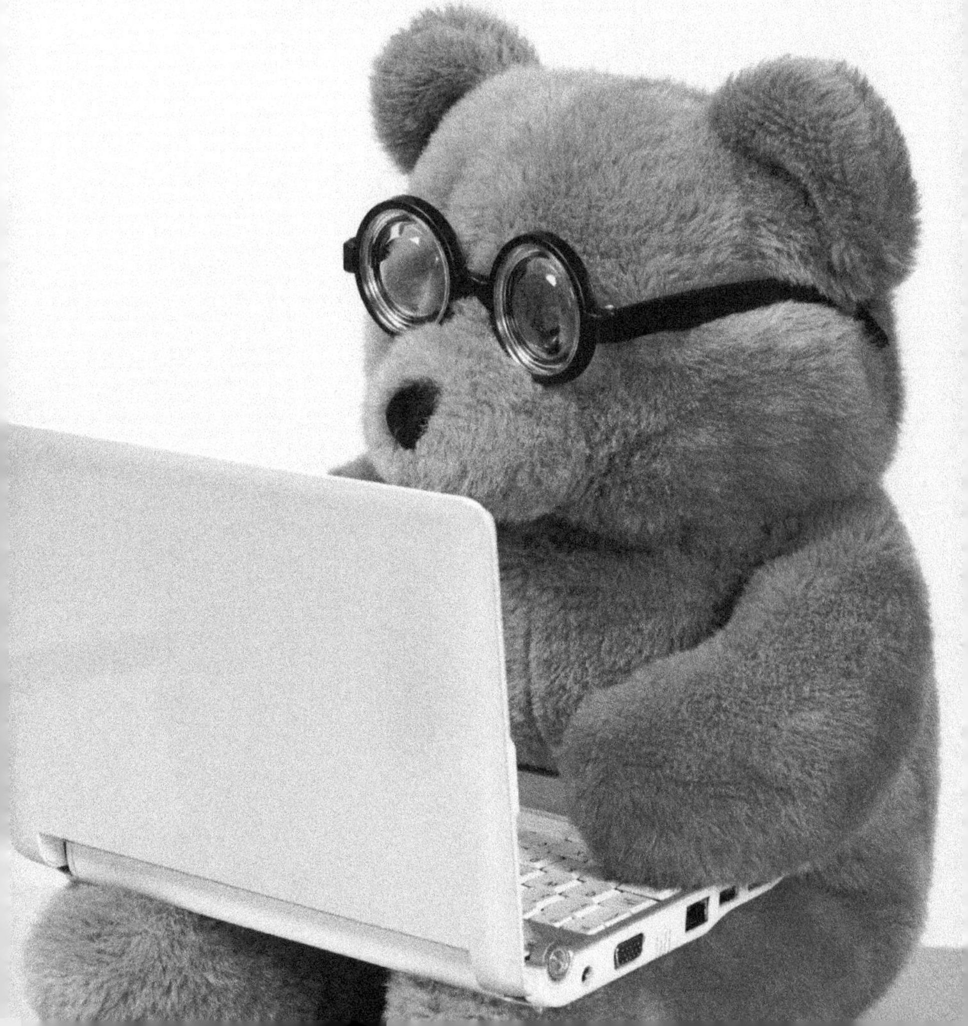

The nursing staff and physician extenders are also vital to your personal experience in the office.

As I walked past the front desk of my office, I heard the calm, low voice of my secretary speaking quietly into the phone.

"Mrs. Atkins, of course we will fit you in to see the doctor, but we don't have an appointment at exactly 3 p.m. Can you come at 4 p.m.?"

A short pause ensued.

"I know Alex's after-school program starts then, but perhaps he could go a little late?"

There was another short pause.

"Yes, I know how important karate is to him, even at four years old."

I continued walking.

The day was busy and filled with a few challenging cases that absorbed my attention. As the afternoon rush in my office began, I heard my secretary raising her voice.

"Ms. Atkins, I know you have been waiting for 15 minutes but you are 30 minutes early for your appointment. I'll be sure to fit you in as soon as we can."

I heard Mrs. Atkins' voice berating my poor secretary. Moments later, my secretary appeared in my office as I finished writing a prescription for another patient.

"Please, Dr. Jones, can you just see her?" my secretary begged me. "She is being so nasty that she is upsetting the rest of the waiting room. I hate to give in to her but she is really creating a scene."

"Of course, Stephanie, please put her in next, just try to be discreet so we don't upset any of the other patients."

Fifteen minutes later I entered the examination room to be met with the warm smile and charming manner of Mrs. Atkins."Oh, doctor, thank you so much for seeing Alex today," she said. "I am just so worried about him."

If I had not just heard the shrill voice of Mrs. Atkins abusing my secretary, I would not have believed this was the same person.

"Thank you so much for fitting us in," she continued. "I called his pediatrician's office and I'm not sure why but the secretary said there was nothing available for a week. Can you imagine? I even tried the pediatrician at our country house in Westchester, and they couldn't see us for two weeks. I'm just amazed at how busy these doctors are."

It is important to realize that the staff at your pediatrician's office are trying to help you get the care you need for your child, from calling for your first appointment to routine interactions. They have a difficult job and we as physicians realize that our office staff is a reflection on our practice. That being said, these usually-young people are only human. If you are disrespectful to them, it makes it more difficult for them to do their jobs.

The old adage that you "catch more flies with honey than vinegar" is especially important as you establish a relationship with the office staff.

One of my favorite families comes frequently to the

office. I have taken care of Mrs. David's children for years and she always takes the time to get to know my staff. She arrives with a small bag of cookies or candies and is always thoughtful about asking about my staff members' lives and children. She is a naturally kind and caring person and I can tell the staff goes out of their way to save an extra lollipop or a special toy for her children. When she mentioned a few years ago that her husband was laid off, it was my secretary's suggestion that I treat her for free until they could get back on their feet.

Contrarily, if you begin your conversation on an adversarial note, it will make it more likely you will receive the same in return. Just remember that at 5:30 p.m. on a Friday night, when you have come home from work and the day care or nanny mentions your child has a fever of 102 degrees, do you want the secretary to say, "Sure, we would be happy to fit you in, run over now," or perhaps you might hear, "So sorry, the doctor is completely booked. Why don't you bring little Jimmy to the emergency room? I'm sure they will see you."

The nursing staff and physician extenders are also vital to your personal experience in the office. After interacting with the front desk staff, your next interaction will most likely be with a physician extender. These support personnel are vital to helping medical offices work efficiently. Support personnel may include medical assistants, scribes, registered nurses, nurse practitioners and physician's assistants. Each one has a specific function in the office and is there to make your experience as stress-free as possible, but most importantly, to care for your child. You have every right to know an individual's name, title and function in the office. It is impossible in this day and age to enter a medical office and not be cared for on some level by physician extenders. If you strongly prefer to only deal with a physician, research concierge practices that will be better equipped to handle that level of personalized care.

Medical assistant: The function of the medical assistant is to help you and your child settle into the exam room, and help you change your child's clothes if necessary. They will routinely take vital signs such as weight, height, blood pressure, temperature, and help collect urine samples if required. In some offices, they also take an initial medical history, answer phone calls, respond to questions after your consultation with your physician, or draw blood samples. Your positive interaction with medical assistants can make your experience in the exam room much better.

Medical scribes: A scribe is a relatively new addition to medical offices, serving as an administrative assistant to the physician. The scribe's responsibility is solely to document your child's encounter in your physician's office. He or she will meet you in the exam room, perform an initial history intake and enter that information into your child's electronic medical record. They will accompany the physician during his or her interview and physical examination of your child before entering that information into your child's chart.

Registered nurse (RN): A registered nurse—often referred to as an "RN"—will assist the physician in caring for your child. They are authorized to administer medication, shots and vaccinations, as well as perform other invasive procedures such as passing a catheter into the bladder to collect a urine specimen, and draw blood. They can administer breathing treatments such as a nebulizer treatment for children with asthma, and in some practices, registered nurses will remove sutures and dress wounds if needed.

Nurse practitioner (NP): The nurse practitioner is the ultimate physician extender, whose primary function in a pediatric office is to act in a supervised but independent role. NPs have advanced training after they receive their RN degree, and hold either a master's or doctorate degree. Each state has different laws requiring the amount of supervision of an NP by a physician. In some states, a nurse practitioner may practice independently from a physician. The American Association of Nurse Practitioners website details state laws and regulations that govern the activity of NP in each state.

Physician's assistant (PA): The physician's assistant has a similar role in the office to a nurse practitioner as a physician extender. Similar to NPs, they can examine, diagnose, treat, and prescribe medication to patients. State law dictates they are required to practice under the supervision of a physician, so their hours are usually similar to their supervising physician.

Your interactions with an NP or PA should be similar

to your interactions with your pediatrician. Many parents will develop therapeutic alliances with the PA or NP over the physicians in the practice. Rest assured if there were a life-threatening condition that develops in your child, the PA, NP and your physician would work together as a team to render the highest level of care.

Fig. 1 (pg 244) details the different roles each health-care provider (NP, PA and MD) have in the office setting.

Chapter 5

Emergencies

How to deal with people you need help from

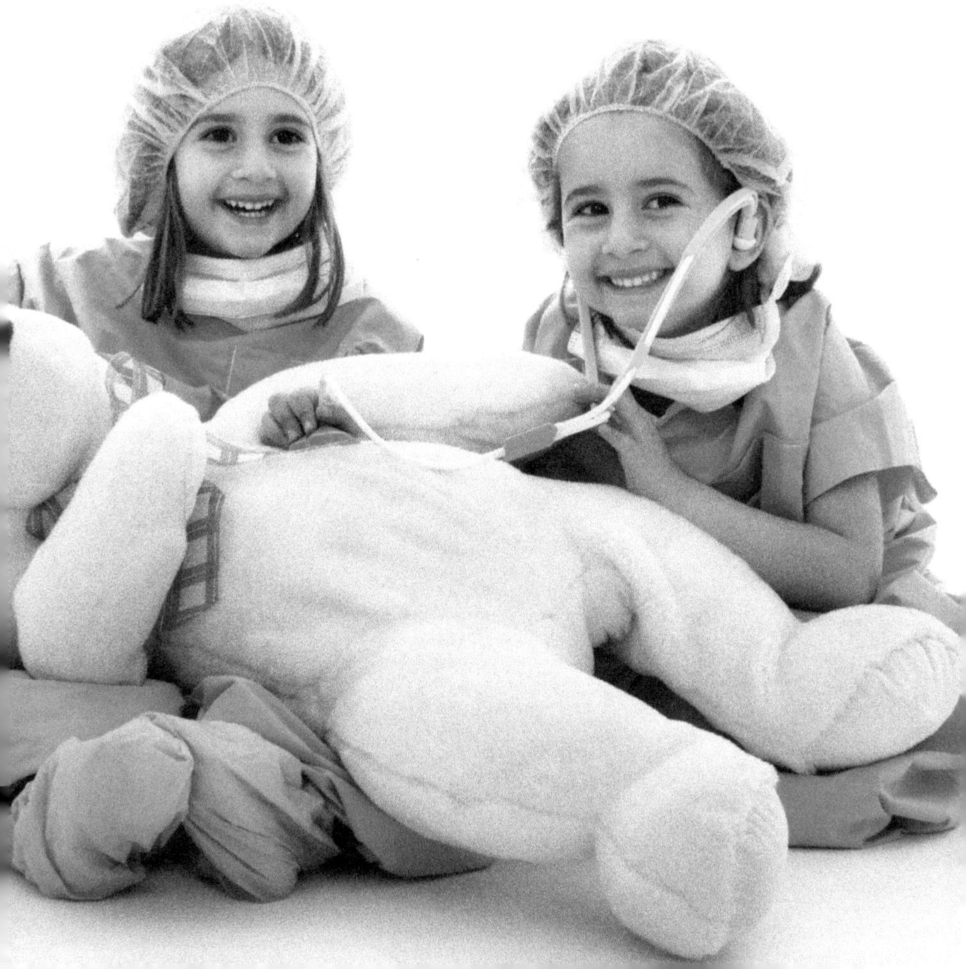

Emergencies are just that: unplanned events that necessitate immediate action on your part.

I lay sprawled on my bed. My body was exhausted. It took great effort to open my eyes. The relentless hacking cough from the room next door invaded the sleep I had embraced just moments before, and awakened me. I tried to raise my body to an upright position as a hand extended over my arm and the deep voice of my husband penetrated my consciousness.

"I'll go," he said. "You must be exhausted."

"Call me if it gets worse," I said. "I'll just rest for a few minutes."

I closed my eyes and allowed the blank curtain of sleep to descend upon me once again.

The past two days had been a battle. My usually happy and easy baby, my second son, had been battling a cold with a flare in his asthma for the past several days. His symptoms seemed relentless. Every two-hour nebulizer, steaming, and the constant need to be held had afforded me little sleep. Thankfully it was a weekend, and my time could be devoted entirely to concentrating on my child. We had been to the pediatrician's office and she had given us explicit instructions on how to manage his illness. I had dealt with many children with asthma and I felt confident that I could manage this crisis on my own.

A shooting pain in my arm woke me up yet again. I

had fallen asleep in an awkward position and my body was protesting the strain I had been inflicting upon myself. As I repositioned myself, I listened closely to my child's breathing, hoping to hear the sounds indicating his progress toward health. The wet, gurgling sound of mucus passing over his swollen vocal cords assailed my senses. The change during just the few hours that I had been sleeping was dramatic. Each breath sounded labored and his wheezing was audible from my bed, fifty feet or more from his crib.

I bolted from my room and rushed towards my sleeping child. My husband lay cradled with our baby in his arms. He was usually calm and nonchalant in his interactions with the children, but that night he looked ashen and worried. "I have tried everything," he said. "He really seems pretty uncomfortable."

I looked down at my son and saw the look of exhaustion on his small face as he struggled to breathe through the thick layers of mucus that closed his throat and lungs.

"Take him into the shower right away and I'll call the pediatrician," I barked to my husband. "We are going to the hospital."

Snapping into physician mode, I struggled into pants and a top as I grabbed the phone, frantically dialing the pediatrician's number. I explained to the answering service that I needed to speak to the doctor immediately, and described the situation at hand as clearly as my trembling voice allowed me to.

Within minutes, the calm voice of my pediatrician reverberated in my ears. "Not to worry Jackie, I agree, it is time to bring him over to the emergency room. Everything's going to be fine. I was on my way into the hospital anyway. I'll meet you there."

I grabbed my wallet and the baby, wrapping him tightly in a warm blanket. My husband called our babysitter to come and care for our older child, who slept with the peace of innocence in his bed next to his brother. The cab deposited me at the emergency entrance of the hospital.

Automatic doors flung open as I strode purposefully to the triage staff of the nurses' station. The nurse rose quickly and—with minimal exchange of information—whisked my son into a treatment room. The residents and attending physicians started a speedy assessment at once. My pediatrician arrived several minutes later and hurried into the room. Within 30 minutes, I was also ushered into the room.

My pediatrician assured me that they had stabilized my son's breathing and that I could sit with him as he slept. The steady beeping of the monitors and bubbling of the oxygen was a comforting yet terrifying sound at the same time. Exhaustion had overtaken him and he lay huddled in the corner of the crib, his small chest rising and falling in a noisy-yet-rhythmic pattern. I descended into a chair and reached through the bars of the crib to hold his small hand as he slumbered.

Emergencies are just that: unplanned events that necessitate immediate action on your part. Your judgment as a parent during these times of crisis can have long-lasting implications upon your child's health.

What constitutes an emergency? It is vital as a consumer of the health-care system to understand which events trigger the emergency system. During the first few weeks as a parent, each sneeze, each cough, each episode of a change in bowel habits is concerning as you navigate the responsibilities of caring for this helpless individual who has captured your heart. Spend time with your pediatrician during your first few visits to understand the warning signs that necessitate an emergency call.

The American Academy of Pediatrics recommends that during the first 12 weeks of life, a fever of 100.4 F (38.0 C) or higher necessitates a call to your pediatrician. In any age child that has a fever that rises above 104 F (40 C) repeatedly, contact your pediatrician right away. If your child is younger than two years old and their fever persists longer than 24 hours or in children over 2 years old with fever over 72 hours in duration, call your pediatrician. If your child has a bad sore throat, ear pain or a rash a call to your pediatrician's office is appropriate.

In any child with significant vomiting and diarrhea that does not improve contact your primary care provider's office for advice.

Signs of dehydration in older children can include a dry diaper or dark yellow urine that is low in quantity.

By now, you have followed instructions to establish your relationship with the office staff. Receiving advice from the nursing staff and ensuring you are in contact with your pediatrician during this period will decrease the possibility of a worsening situation. Make sure that all of the adults involved in your child's care understand the warning signs that your pediatrician discussed with you, which require a change in your care plan.

After-hours calls to your health-care provider: The majority of pediatric offices will be open Monday to Friday from 9 a.m. to 5 p.m. Larger providers may have weekend hours for sick visits. It is important during your initial visits to establish a plan with your health-care provider on how to handle after-hours calls. After-hours calls will in most cases be directed to an answering service. These individuals are not medical professionals, and just as 9-1-1 operators do, receive training on how to triage calls.

As you interact with an answering service, it is important to stay calm and impart as much vital information as possible so that a health-care provider who knows how urgent your situation is can be contacted. Remember, the answering service will not have access to your child's record, so do not become frustrated if they ask you a series of questions such as name, date of birth and the best number to reach you. Be sure to have your local pharmacy number available to give the answering service or physician when they call back, if in the best situation, your child can be cared for at home.

Think of the symptoms that concern you and let the answering service know. Try to keep it short, to ensure that your top concerns are relayed to the physician on call. Otherwise, your call could be put lower down on the priority list and may delay response time.

Try this: "Johnny is 1 year old and has been vomiting for over 24 hours. His diaper is dry."

Not this: "We went to a friend's house with Johnny three days ago. He seemed cranky there but I ignored it, and yesterday, we went to the market. You know that one on Third Avenue. They have the best breadsticks. Oh he just loves these breadsticks and wouldn't eat one. I wasn't really concerned but then last night, he wouldn't take his bottle. I tried multiple times. This morning when I woke him up, he just wasn't himself…"

Once your information has been given to the service, stay off the phone. Be sure to disable any call screening features so that your pediatrician can call you back. Call your telephone carrier after your initial pediatric visit to find out what blocking features are present on your phone.

If you have not heard back from a health-care provider within 20 minutes, call the service again and let them know this is your second call and that they should try and reach your pediatrician via another route.

When a health-care provider calls back, they may or may not have access to your child's records so it is important to share with them significant health concerns such as allergies to medications, or what medications or interventions you have been using to treat your child's illness. Have a pen and paper ready to jot down notes, and your pharmacy number if medication needs to be prescribed. Make sure prior to placing a call to your primary care provider's office that your pharmacy is open and that your child is registered with the pharmacy.

Nursing services: Some practices will have their calls triaged to a nursing service. Registered nurses who are experienced in pediatric emergency care answer these emergency calls. They are trained to escalate your concerns to a covering pediatrician and advise you to call 9-1-1 in life-threatening situations. The vast majority of these practitioners are well trained and it is likely you will receive excellent care from them. Discuss any concerns you may have regarding interacting with these nursing services with your pediatrician at a routine office visit.

Urgent care centers: In many parts of the country, urgent care centers are springing up on street corners, malls, and even some pharmacies. It is important to research these facilities prior to your needing them. Are the health-care providers physicians or physician extenders? Do they treat children, and if so, what training does the staff have in dealing with pediatric emergencies? Take time to discuss with your pediatrician their thoughts on the local urgent care centers. There will most likely be urgent care centers they have worked with in the past, and can recommend.

Local emergency rooms may also have urgent care facilities and may have a pediatrician on call to staff these facilities. If you feel uncomfortable with the advice or care you have received from any freestanding urgent care center, a call to your pediatrician or a visit to your local emergency room is advisable.

When to call 9-1-1: Your pediatrician/primary care provider can only offer a limited amount of emergency services in their office. If you have concerns about a life-threatening emergency, call 9-1-1. If your child is struggling to breathe and rapidly worsening, and if they appear unresponsive or their lips are turning a bluish color, then emergency help is needed. A seizure, excessive bleeding, or loss of consciousness following a fall are warning signs that immediate emergency help is needed.

Stay calm and have one parent stay with the child while the other calls 9-1-1. It is extremely difficult to remain entirely calm in a life-threatening situation that involves your child, but your child's life may depend on your focused action during this critical time. When the paramedics arrive, bring any medication your child has been taking with you and decide which parent will ride with your child in the ambulance. Whichever parent is the calmest should ride with the paramedics. Paramedics will bring your child to the closest possible emergency room. The most important factor to consider is that there will be capable professionals dealing with the emergency. Be sure to alert your pediatrician as to which hospital your child will be taken to. Once your child is stabilized, you and your pediatrician may feel transfer to another facility is indicated and they can start the process of arranging for a transfer to a hospital of your choice.

As with all emergencies, having a plan in place that you and your pediatrician agree on will make it less likely that your child will require the urgent transfer to the hospital via ambulance. Taking time at your routine visit to discuss your emergency preparedness plan with your pediatrician will decrease the stress on both of you during these critical times in your child's health.

Chapter 6
Referral to a Specialist

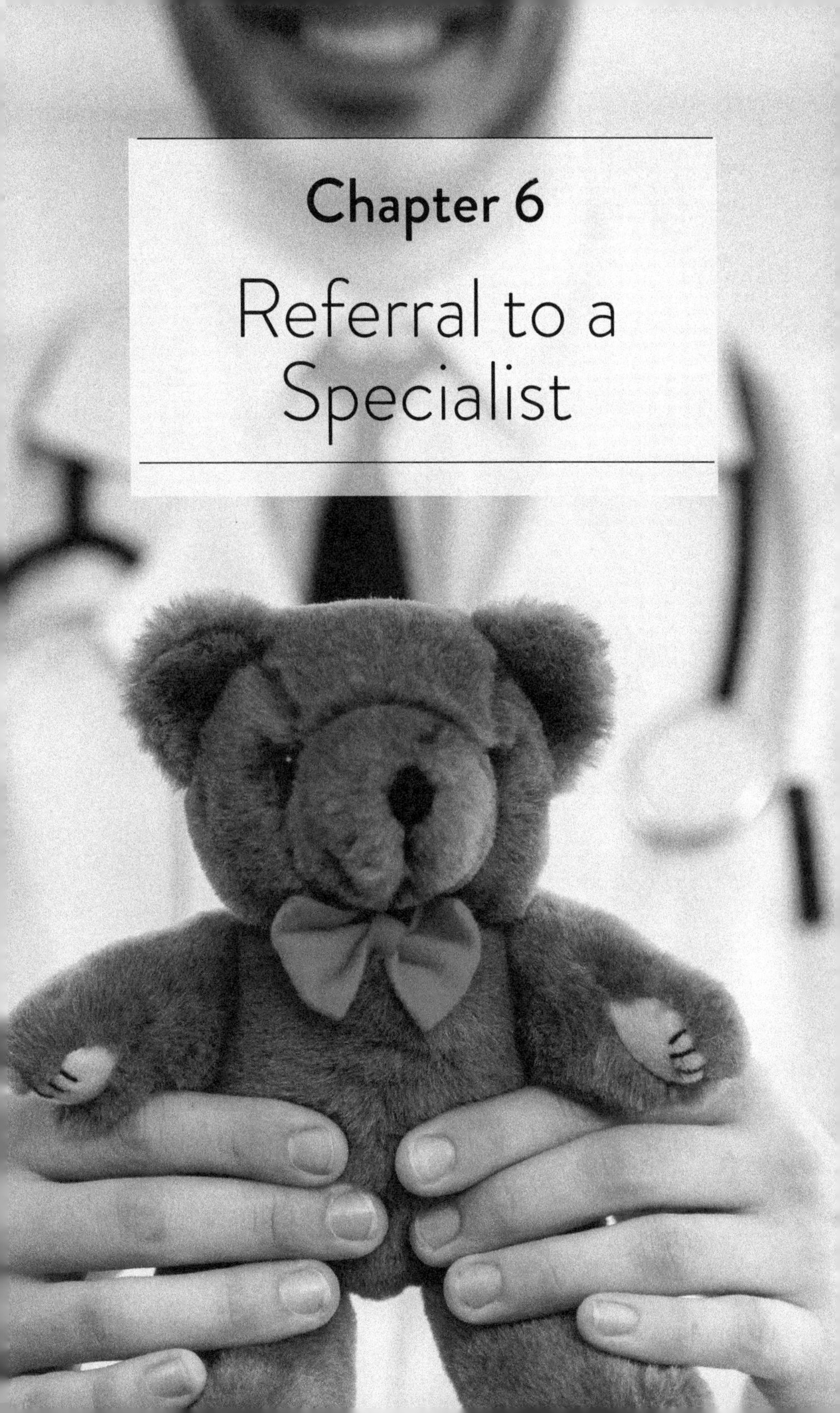

Specialization allows a physician to concentrate on an area of medicine in their field.

I fidgeted on the hard bench in the reception area, waiting to be called into my pediatrician's office, and gazing at the sleeping child in my arms. Just one week earlier, we had been sitting under the cold fluorescent light of the emergency room, as he struggled to breathe. Hours of nebulizers and steroids only made him restless and irritable during the days to follow, consuming much of my waking hours. I was frazzled and needed the reassurance that my pediatrician always brought to our conversations.

"Dr. Jones, please follow me," the medical assistant murmured and smiled warmly. "The doctor will see you now."

I rose stiffly carrying the sleeping bundle in my arms. I carefully laid him down on the exam table and tried to slowly peel the clothes from his chunky body. The mucous rattling in his chest had become a constant backdrop to his rhythmic breathing. The efforts of the past week had taken their toll on us both. He slept as I moved him from side to side, gingerly removing his clothes.

The door opened and my pediatrician arrived. Her gentle manner was a sharp contrast to the anxiety I felt, as I listened to the gurgle of mucous that emanated from my child. We propped the baby up and the doctor listened carefully to his lungs and neck. I could tell by the amount of time she spent on his right side that she was unhappy with her findings.

"Jackie, his lungs are better, but I'm still a little concerned," she said. "I think it's time we had him see a lung specialist."

The idea of a specialist made the situation seem much more serious. It was something that I was not ready to accept.

"Perhaps if we just try some antibiotics it will all go away," I replied, knowing that this suggestion was not getting to the root of the underlying problem.

"No," the physician responded. "I think he might need antibiotics, but I'd like to figure out a longer term plan to keep him out of the emergency room in the future."

Trips to the ER, nebulizers and steroids were all indications that a specialist was the best course of action. I just needed to accept that my child needed more help.

The advances in medicine over the past 50 years have been astonishing. From our ability to keep 28-week, premature infants alive, to our triumphs in the fight against cancer, the amount of specialized information a physician must assimilate to be the best in every field is overwhelming. Specialization allows a physician to concentrate on an area of medicine in their field, and the rapid changes and progressions within it. Consultation with a specialist will afford you and your primary care physician the opportunity to receive an expert opinion on the best course of treatment for your child.

Choosing a specialist: In most cases, your primary care provider will refer you to a specialist. Location, hospital affiliation, and—if needed—insurance participation are all factors that may influence your pediatrician's recommendations. Most primary care providers work with several specialists, who share similar treatment styles and philosophies. Ask for two or three names so that you have options when it comes to choosing an individual who is right for you.

It is vital that you and your primary care physician discuss which issues they feel are important for the specialist to address, and in what time frame you should see the specialist. Ask your pediatrician to write down a brief history that you can bring with you. They should list the issues they would like the specialist to address. Read over the note with your pediatrician so that you understand your child's medical history and what the purpose of the consultation is.

Do your research before seeing the specialist by checking their hospital affiliations, browsing their website, and checking online reviews to get a sense of their reputation in the community. National referral sites—such as Castle and Connolly's Top Doctors list—can be reputable sources of additional information. Ask friends and neighbors which specialists they have worked with and if they were happy with their visits. In smaller communities, there may be only one or two choices for specialists. You must decide if you feel comfortable with those choices or if you prefer to travel to a larger area to receive a different consultation.

Scheduling your visit: Getting a sense of how urgent the visit is from your primary care provider will be important when it comes to scheduling your appointment. If the situation requires an emergent visit, ask your pediatrician's office to call on your behalf, and they should let the specialist know you will be calling and that the pediatrician would appreciate your being fit in as soon as possible. Demanding an emergency appointment for a less urgent matter may affect how seriously your requests for follow-up appointments are taken in the future. Be flexible in your request for an appointment if you truly need your child seen right away.

If the office is fitting you in, be prepared for there to be a wait and decide if you are okay with that, or if you want to try another provider. Collect as much information as you can that may be helpful for the consultant. The more information that you can provide at the initial evaluation, the better the advice you will receive.

Try to condense that information into a manageable form for review during your visit. Thirty pages of medical records as well as X-rays and pharmacy records will make it impossible for the consultant to adequately review all of the information and make an educated assessment for you at the time of your visit.

Specialty visits: A specialist may be required to perform additional testing that your pediatrician may not have the ability to perform in their office. This may range from non-invasive testing, such as a hearing test or an EKG, to more invasive testing such as an endoscopy (a scope used to look into spaces that can not be easily examined) or a catheterization (a small tube used to obtain urine for evaluation). When making the appointment, inquire about additional charges.

When meeting the specialist, you will have the opportunity to discuss your concerns and your primary care provider's concerns. Be as concise as possible in sharing your child's medical history and tell the specialist what you are looking to get out of the visit. If your spouse/significant other is unable to attend the appointment with you, ask if they can join the visit via phone. The specialist may or may not have access to your child's medical history, so be patient in sharing this information with them. Other important information that they might need includes your child's birth history, any significant illnesses, as well as hospitalizations or surgery since birth. Be sure to share any family history of diseases that are related to your child's current problem. Many diseases have a genetic component and it is helpful for the specialist to understand how both parents' medical history may be reflected in their child's current medical condition. If medications have been used to treat your child's medical condition, bring a list of those and the dates they were used. You can contact your pharmacy for a list of the medications your child has received.

If you are seeing the specialist about a rash or any problem you have been noticing visually, bring pictures of the progression of the problem. If you are seeing the doctor about snoring or problems breathing, bring an audiotape of several minutes duration of your child's breathing. If your child is seeing a therapist for behavioral problems such as temper tantrums, a videotape of the concerning behavior is helpful.

After you have shared your child's history and answered all the physician's questions, discuss what the physical examination portion of the exam will entail. Decide if your child needs to be restrained for any portion of the exam and who will do that. In many cases, both the medical staff and a parent are needed to make sure your child does not move during critical portions of the evaluation. Being forthcoming with your concerns or anxiety about the exam is helpful so that you and your specialist can start to develop a relationship.

It is ultimately your decision what test you want to have performed. Prohibiting the physician from gathering information may hamper their ability to provide an accurate diagnosis and recommendations. Be respectful of your child. Don't ask them if they will allow a procedure to be performed if you have decided to go ahead with the procedure. If they say no are you willing to conclude the examination at that point? Spending half an hour negotiating with a two-year-old so the specialist can look into their mouth is not an effective use of your time or the specialist's time, and sends the wrong message to your child if you ultimately proceed with the examination.

Be sure to take notes and ask for diagrams when discussing findings with the physician. This is your opportunity to become educated in the issues of your child's medical condition from a specialist. As the specialist makes their recommendations, ask if there are any alternatives to the course of therapy they have suggested. Inquire if additional testing is required before a definitive diagnosis can be made or if medication is indicated at this visit. If medication is indicated, ask which problem will it be treating and how will it work to improve the condition. Inquire how the medication is administered and what potential side effects there are. Ask how long the medication will be administered and when you and your child should follow up.

Follow-up appointments: Most specialists will require a follow-up appointment to discuss the results of any testing that may have been performed and to check the progress of your child's condition. At your initial visit, set up a time frame for how long it will take the specialist to obtain results of any testing, and how the results of that testing will be conveyed to you. Will the results be reported over the phone or should you make an appointment to visit the specialist? If the results will be delivered over the phone, will the physician be calling to discuss the results or will a nurse or another physician extender be calling? It can be anxiety-provoking to wait for results, but realize if you rush the interpretation of those results, you may not have the best person interpreting them.

I occasionally get requests from parents asking for immediate results from a radiology test. Rushing the process may alleviate your anxiety but may not allow you access to the most experienced opinion available. While I understand why a parent would want immediate results, that request does not leave me enough time to contact a radiologist to review the films. In many situations, physicians have a radiologist they know and trust, and would prefer waiting for them to interpret the results. In life-threatening situations, whoever is on call will read the films.

I strongly recommend discussing test results in person. A call from your physician to come to the office to discuss results should take precedence over almost any other activity you have planned. I distinctly remember receiving results from a routine surgical specimen that surprisingly showed evidence of cancer in a six-year-old. I called the mother and father and asked them to come in that day, but they were very busy and really didn't want to take time off work. The more I pushed the more they pushed back until I had no choice but to discuss the results with them over the phone so we could move forward with the appropriate referrals and treatment.

Delivering that sort of information over the phone was stressful for me and devastating for them. I could not look into their eyes and assure them I would do everything I could to help them work through this problem. It is also important for parents to be together upon receiving concerning information in order to support each other.

Luckily, most times I am not dealing with such dire news, but the results of testing do help me to formulate a treatment plan and make recommendations moving forward to address my patient's illness and their parents' concerns. I encourage parents to take notes during our visit and to use my website as a resource. I try to include on my website information about the more common problems I encounter and some of the options for treatment.

Follow-up visits are great opportunities to get a feel for your specialist's personality and their style of medicine. Do they clearly discuss the results? What are the implications of these findings?

Do they educate you on the anatomy and physiology of the problem you are dealing with? Are they patient with you as you process this information and work through the options available? Do they give you at least two options for treatment of the problem (if possible) and do they clearly discuss the advantages and disadvantages of these options?

The internet: The internet is a resource like no other in that the amount of information a health-care consumer can obtain is overwhelming—but therein lies the problem. There is no filter on the information and much of it may not apply to your child's unique medical condition. Your primary care provider and specialist should be the ones supplying you with the bulk of the information concerning your child's medical condition. Take the time to discuss any information you have found online, but remember that you came to your specialist for their recommendations and guidance. Thus, trying to formulate your own treatment plan from information you have obtained from the internet is not in your child's best interest.

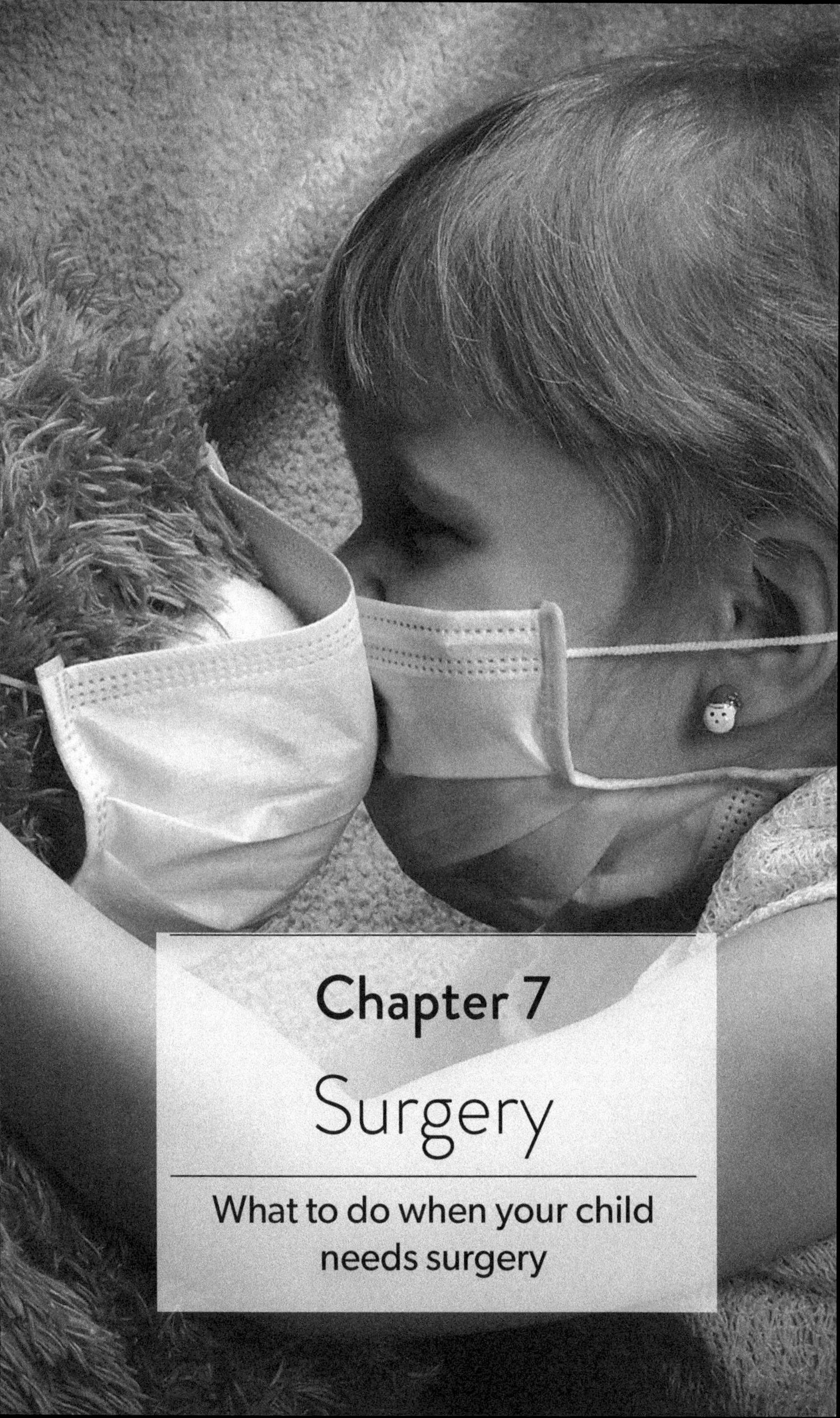

Chapter 7

Surgery

What to do when your child needs surgery

In great detail, she described the anatomic concerns and why she thought it was appropriate that our pediatrician had referred us to her. With diagrams and handouts, she went step-by-step through her findings and our concerns.

My one-year-old son squirmed under the probing fingers of the pediatrician. We had both noticed, soon after birth, that the normal symmetry of his testes was absent. On one side of his groin, there was a small pea-shaped bulge that housed his undescended testicle. Although this did not constitute an emergency, leaving the testicle inside the body could lead to infertility and more serious problems later in life. She examined him thoroughly then turned to me with her thoughts.

"It doesn't seem to have moved," she said. "We should probably have him see the pediatric urologist. There are several very talented surgeons. Let's get their opinions."

At the top of the list of names that she handed to me was a young surgeon who had started at New York-Presbyterian around the same time I had. Personable and friendly, she struck me as a nice person. Next on the list was the chairman of the department of urology for one of the most esteemed programs in the city. Well-regarded and accomplished in his field, he was my first choice. I called his office the following morning to schedule an appointment, using all my powers of persuasion to obtain one for a long two weeks ahead. On the day of the appointment, I arrived early with my first-born son clutched tightly to my chest. He was one of those babies who preferred his independence to the tight embrace I offered. As soon as we entered the play area, he was out of my arms exploring the brightly colored toys scattered about the floor. My husband arrived soon thereafter and was a calming relief to my nervous energy.

Within an hour, we were ushered into an exam room where we were met by a nurse who handed me a small gown to place on my wriggling son. We waited another 20 minutes before the door swung open, and a young man dressed in the traditional rumpled green scrubs of residency greeted us. He took a detailed history and examined my child, who was now beginning to lose his spirit of cooperation and protested vehemently to the poking and prodding in his diaper area. The young doctor told us that he concurred with our pediatrician's findings of an undescended testis and informed us the chairman would be in soon. Another 20 minutes passed and, thankfully, my son had reached his limit. He sat curled up in my lap clutching his teddy to his small chest.

The door swung open and the larger-than-life personality of the chairman consumed the room.

"Well hello there, sweetheart," he boomed at me, each word dripping with southern twang. "So nice to meet you. Now, who might these attractive young men be?"

My mouth dropped open as I struggled to extend my hand and I glanced quickly around the room to make sure he was speaking to me. I had not been called "sweetheart" since I became a physician seven years ago. I stammered an introduction of my husband and sleeping son.

"Well, why don't you take the pants off that fine young

man so I can examine him," the doctor said. "The sleeping one I mean," he chuckled, and winked at my husband.

A Bostonian for too many generations to count, my husband's body tighten as his arm rested gently against me.

I jumped up, fearing a confrontation, and quickly undressed my son. The doctor examined him and discussed his findings and thought process with the resident, standing closely beside him. He quickly reattached my screaming and overtired son's diaper and stepped back as I scooped my child into my arms.

"Well, it definitely looks like that testis has not come down," he said. "Let's go ahead and get him set up for surgery. My nurse will be back in a few minutes to give you all the details."

He turned toward the door and began his exit from the room.

"Excuse me, doctor," I bellowed over the screaming of my wriggling son. "Would you mind explaining the indications for surgery and how it will be performed?"

He turned and looked at me with the exasperated air one might give to a child who asked why the sky was blue.

"Pretty straightforward," he said. "If we don't operate, he has a high chance of being sterile. I have done thousands of these. Trust me, I'll do a wonderful job."

He smiled benevolently at me and strode from the room. As the exam room door closed, my husband rose.

"Jackie, I think it's time to go. I don't think this is the right fit," he said.

I hesitated before responding.

"He's done thousands of these," I murmured. "That's worth a lot, you know."

"Jackie," he said. "I don't think it's the right fit. Let's go."

I knew my husband was right, and I quickly dressed our son before hurrying down the hall and into the elevator behind my husband.

The next morning I called the young surgeon recommended by my pediatrician. She agreed to see us the following afternoon. We were quickly escorted into her office by one of the nurses bypassing the crowded waiting room. In less than 30 minutes, we were escorted into the brightly-lit exam room. I placed my young son on the examination table as the door swung open.

"Jackie, it's so nice to see you and I'm honored that you have brought your son in," the physician said. Her warm smile radiated confidence and a calm demeanor—both things I needed to combat my anxiety about the discussion that lay ahead. The doctor performed a thorough medical history and physical examination, before giving my son a tongue depressor to play with as she sat down to discuss her recommendations.

"Since I understand you're not a physician," she said, turning toward my husband, "let me take some time to go over the anatomy and discuss my findings."

In great detail, she described the anatomic concerns and why she thought it was appropriate that our pediatrician had referred us to her. With diagrams and handouts, she went step-by-step through her findings and our concerns.

"While the testes has not completely descended, I feel

that it is starting to move and I would recommend us reexamining him in three months," she said. "If the testes have not completely descended by that time, let's proceed with surgery."

I'm not sure if my sigh of relief was audible, but I felt a huge weight had been lifted from my shoulders. I reached for my husband's hand and felt his reassuring squeeze as I smiled. I thanked the doctor for her time, and she encouraged me to call any time should more concerns arise.

As the latch to the door snapped into place, my husband rose. "Well that was better," he said. "I think I understand the problem now. Let's hope for the best."

Choosing your surgeon: A surgeon is a specialist who performs surgery, and choosing one for your child is one of the most difficult decisions you will make as you navigate the health-care system with your child.

You should use the same criteria to evaluate surgeons as you would a medical specialist: Your pediatrician's referral, referrals from family and friends, as well as the internet and national referral websites.Surgery is a technical field, so obtaining information about where the surgeon completed their residency and fellowship are also important. These residency and fellowship programs will be ranked in national and international publications based on the quality of the program. All information obtained from the internet must be taken in the context it is reported.

For example, learning that your surgeon trained at a hospital that has a higher complication rate than a surgeon who trained at a smaller hospital may be concerning on first glance. However, that larger hospital may take care of sicker patients and may not have the same rates of success as a community hospital with a healthier population. These larger hospitals may also have higher rates of complications than a community hospital as they have sicker patients. However, their trainees may have graduated with extensive operative experience and know how to take care of any complication that may arise.

Research your child's condition prior to your visit with the surgeon. Get an idea of what options may be available to treat your child's illness and if surgery is the only option. Make a list of questions and make sure that your spouse or significant other will be available for the visit. If you share custody of your child with a parent who does not live with you, discuss how you will make the decision prior to the visit. Bickering in a physician's office is not helpful to the physician and can be extremely anxiety provoking for your child.

Have your surgeon go through the reasons why they are recommending surgery. Discuss the anatomy and how surgery will help to address your child's medical problem. Don't be afraid to ask questions and if other options are available.

Be sure to discuss complications and what the process of recovery will entail:

- How long will your child be in the hospital if that is indicated?

- How long will they need to be out of daycare or school?
- How long should you or your spouse be home from work?
- This is an excellent time to get a feeling for how supportive your surgeon will be during this stressful process. When explaining the surgery, are they patient and informative, or dismissive and rushed?

If you do not understand what is said to you, be sure to stop and ask for a more detailed explanation. You will be asked to sign a consent form indicating that you have discussed the surgery with your surgeon, and understand the risks and benefits. Be sure that the procedure is listed and the site of the surgery is indicated on the consent form, and that your family and the surgeon agree on exactly what type of surgery is being performed. If you have questions about the consent form or type of surgery to be performed, discuss them with your surgeon prior to surgery. The day of surgery is not the time to have an in-depth discussion about alternatives to surgery or changes to the surgical procedure, as your surgeon will be preparing for the surgery, and you, as parents, will be nervous and not thinking clearly.

A good pediatric surgery office is aware of a family's anxiety around surgery, and will make themselves available to help manage that anxiety.

Preparing yourself and your child for surgery: Several studies indicate that a parent's emotional state is directly correlated to those of their child's before and after surgery. A study in the *Journal of Paediatrics and Child Health* found that children between ages two and five years whose parents were more anxious prior to surgery also had a higher level of anxiety than children whose parents were less anxious.[3] An article in The Journal of Pain found that children whose parent's catastrophize their child's pain preoperatively had greater pain intensity postoperatively than those whose parents did not.[4] In parental catastrophizing, a parent will tend to describe their child's pain in more exaggerated terms and dwell on the pain or illness more than other parents.

Be cognizant of what you discuss in front of your child about their upcoming surgery. They are able to comprehend more than we give them credit for. Before discussing the surgery with the doctor or nurse, send children older than five years old to the office's play area. It is the parent's responsibility to discuss the upcoming surgery with their child once they have made their decision. Young children can only process a limited amount of information prior to surgery. I recommend letting children know two or three days prior to surgery that they will be visiting the hospital so their doctor can make them feel better.

Many surgical facilities will require a visit to your primary care provider prior to surgery. This preoperative visit is a wonderful opportunity to discuss your child's upcoming surgery and talk through any concerns you might have with your primary care provider. They can also give you advice and help navigate the process of preparing your child for surgery. Discuss if or how your primary care provider will be involved in your child's care following the surgery, if they are being admitted overnight to the hospital. During this visit, your primary care provider will also examine your child and possibly perform blood work to forward to the surgeon. This information is commonly reviewed by the nursing and anesthesia staff prior to surgery so any medical concerns that might impact your child's surgery can be addressed preoperatively.

Larger hospitals may have preoperative programs available for you and your child to help prepare for surgery. These programs consist of a visit to the hospital or ambulatory care facility prior to surgery, where you and your child meet with a child life specialist or another member of the health-care team to go through a step-by-step process outlining the events that will take place on the day of the surgery. They may use dolls and videos, which are age appropriate, to answer questions you and your child may have. The two biggest fears that children have prior to surgery, in my experience, are that parents will leave them and that they will get a shot. Pediatric specialists are aware of these fears and will work as a team to minimize the preoperative anxiety you or your child may have.

Surgical facilities: The hospital or facility where your surgeon operates is almost as important a decision as choosing your surgeon. Surgery can be performed at an outpatient facility or inpatient setting, depending on the complexity of the surgery and your child's age. In many settings, children who are under six months old are required to stay overnight. If your child has a chronic or acute illness, or surgery is complex, they also may require overnight admission. If your child is required to stay overnight, your surgeon will provide information on the hospital.

It is also important to discuss which parent will stay overnight with the child postoperatively. In most hospitals, this is a common practice and strongly encouraged. If both parents would like to stay, a private room is required and this will not be covered by insurance in most cases. Ask your surgeon's office for information on availability of a private room and the costs.

The hospital is not a restful environment and if both parents are exhausted, they may not have the resources emotionally and physically to give the child the full attention they may require. I usually encourage one parent to stay in the hospital and the other to go home.

You can check the hospital's website for pictures of a typical pediatric room. Will your child require more specialized care such as an intensive care unit setting? Be sure to ask if parents are allowed to stay if intensive care observation is required.In many institutions, your child will be encouraged to wear hospital pajamas or a gown, so the nurses can easily access their arms and legs to take blood pressures, check surgical dressings, check their intravenous line and listen to their heart and lungs. Bring your child's comfort items (a blanket, teddy bear, etc.), along with comfortable clothes and toiletries for yourself.

It is the nursing staff's job to assure that your child is stable and is receiving the medication the doctors have ordered. Vital signs may be taken every one, four, or six hours as ordered by the physicians. The nursing staff must follow the orders of the physician so arguing with them about waking your child may not be in your child's best interest. Asking questions and understanding why the physicians have requested frequent monitoring will help you feel comfortable with the frequency you and your child are disturbed. In some cases, continuous monitoring will be required and helping your child feel comfortable with the monitors will be a task left to you and the nursing staff.

In larger hospitals, there may be doctors in training such as interns, residents, and fellows. Your child will most likely see both pediatric and surgical doctors in training who assist your physicians to care for your child. In larger hospitals, it is virtually impossible to request that no doctors in training see your child. The interns, residents, and fellows are the workhorses in an academic institution and round with the attending physicians once or twice a day. They are in constant contact with the supervising physicians if there is a significant change in your child's health or if they are critically ill. If you feel you would like care only by an attending physician, look for a smaller, nonacademic hospital and surgeon.

Ambulatory centers: More and more surgeries are being performed in ambulatory surgery centers. These are usually free-standing facilities that are not physically connected to a hospital. The advantages of ambulatory surgery centers are that they are usually very efficiently run with a focus on patient satisfaction. They are commonly staffed with only attending physicians and rarely do physicians in training participate in the care of the patients.

The disadvantages of ambulatory surgery centers are that they cannot do complicated surgeries and they do not have the ability to monitor patients overnight. Some ambulatory surgery centers have extensive experience in caring for children, but it is wise to ask your surgeon if nurses and anesthesiologists who are skilled in the care of children are employed by the facility. Surgeons want patients to be well cared for and safe, but it never hurts to inquire and feel comfortable with your choice.

Pre-surgery guidelines: Your surgeon's office and the hospital will provide you with instructions on medications that need to be avoided prior to surgery. Please be sure to review these carefully, for in some cases, over-the-counter medications and vitamins may need to be discontinued two weeks prior to surgery. You will also receive instructions on when your child should stop eating and drinking prior to surgery. In many facilities, children must refrain from solid food eight hours prior to surgery, milk six hours prior to surgery, breast milk four hours prior to surgery, and clear liquids such as water and apple juice three hours prior to surgery. Each hospital and facility has their own guidelines, so be sure to review them with your surgeon's office and the facility prior to surgery.

Surgery day: Your first medical interactions when you arrive at the hospital or surgery center will be with the nursing staff. They will interview you and sometimes your child if he or she is old enough. They will confirm the information that your pediatrician and surgeon have provided and will review the consent form with you, along with the site of surgery. Be patient with them as it is their job to assure your child's safety. Many different individuals may ask you the same question multiple times to ensure that it is conveyed from you and not just from the written chart. The nursing staff will perform vital signs, and ask your child to change into hospital pajamas—which are sterilized by the facility and allow access to your child during surgery.

It is a good idea to tell your child ahead of the surgery that they will be wearing "special clothes" at the hospital, which often makes the process of changing into them a bit easier. You will be escorted to the operating room by the nursing staff or support staff. In most facilities, one or both parents may come to the operating room with their child, and stay with them as they are put to sleep.

You will be asked to wear a jumpsuit and shoe covers, as well as a hat and mask to avoid contamination of the operating room with dirt and germs from the street. Dress in flat, closed-toe shoes and comfortable clothing. Discussing with your child that mommy and daddy will get to wear a special outfit may help prepare them that you will look different as well.

Once you arrive at the operating room, the nursing staff will escort you inside and you and your child will meet the operating room staff, anesthesia staff, and your surgeon.

Anesthesia: Anesthesia is among the main causes of anxiety for parents with children going into surgery. There are two types of anesthesia—general and local/regional anesthesia. Local/regional anesthesia is similar to what one would receive in a dentist's office. A series of injections of a local anesthetic that will render the area injected numb to pain. This is difficult to perform in younger children as many children have a fear of needles. Local anesthesia can only be used for minor procedures such as the excision of skin lesions and lesions directly under the skin. Surgery on the mouth or airway that need to be protected or in areas such as the eye, where the movement during the procedure could lead to a catastrophe, is also not amenable to local anesthesia.

Regional or spinal anesthesia involves the installation of a local anesthetic into a group of nerves, rendering them numb to pain. In adults, a spinal anesthetic is used to anesthetize the lower body for surgery. This is a difficult process in very young children who often have difficulty sitting still during the application of local anesthetic and, once numb, may not be able to understand why they can't move their legs or arms thus becoming agitated and anxious.

A recent study performed at Columbia Presbyterian Hospital in New York found that children being exposed to anesthetics of short durations (80 minutes or less) had no long-term effect on their intellectual development later in life. The study examined 105 sibling pairs—one underwent hernia repair, the other child did not have surgery or anesthesia. The mean age of the children receiving anesthesia was 17 months of age at the time of surgery and they were tested again at 10 years of age. The study showed no difference in IQ between the children exposed to anesthesia and surgery versus their siblings who were not exposed.[5]

Studies like these help us feel confident in assuring parents that there is no significant risk of long-term issues with brain development later in life from short-term exposure to anesthesia even at a young age.

While anxiety-provoking for parents, the use of general anesthesia is—for many pediatric surgical procedures—the safest choice. The anesthesiologist in consultation with your child's surgeon should ultimately be the one deciding which method of anesthesia to administer.

We, as pediatric surgeons, put together a team we feel comfortable with. This includes nurses, surgical technologists and anesthesiologists. It is fine to discuss whom your surgeon uses and who comprises their team. Asking if a fellowship-trained pediatric anesthesiologist or one with a great deal of pediatric experience is available is absolutely appropriate. However, once you have done your research and have laid your trust in your surgeon and his/her choice of an operating facility, rest assured that they will do their best to ensure the utmost quality from the entire surgical team—therefore try not to interfere in their choices.

Recovery room: Once your child's surgery is complete, you will join them in the recovery room. The majority of children wake up from anesthesia crying and some are combative. This is generally due to the dissociative effects on the brain caused by general anesthesia. I equate it to the feeling of someone slipping you a triple martini and not telling you. Adults wake up dizzy and often don't feel well. We have the ability with our mature brains to understand the feeling will pass. Children do not understand, and instead, tend to scream and cry about the dizzy, sick feeling they are experiencing. The calmer you can be during this phase, the better your child will react.

Anesthesia does have amnestic properties, so it is unlikely children will remember much of this distressing phase. Most children undergoing short procedures of 90 minutes or less will have a disassociated phase that will last for approximately 30 minutes. It is common for children to fall asleep again, but they will wake up feeling better after about a 30-minute nap. Each child's response to anesthesia is unique so take these numbers as a rough guide.

A registered nurse in the post-anesthesia care unit will care for your child. In most facilities, your nurse will have only one to three patients to care for. This assures that you and your child will receive personalized attention.

When the nursing staff feels your child is stable and in compliance with hospital protocol and your physician's orders, your child will be discharged home. You will likely not see your surgeon when you are discharged as they are tending to other patients in the operating room. Rest assured that the nursing professionals who staff the recovery room are skilled in assessing your child. If there is concern, they will contact your child's anesthesiologist and surgeon.

When your child is ready to be discharged, you will receive instructions from your surgeon. Please review these instructions carefully with the nursing staff. Make sure that you understand how to administer your child's postoperative medication. Before you leave, be sure to inquire when the last dose of pain medication was administered so you know when the next dose should be given. If your child vomits easily, ask for disposable large towels to take with you for your car ride home.Unless this is an extremely minor procedure that did not require anesthesia, public transportation is not advisable. If possible, try not to be alone in the car driving your child home, as you may be distracted checking on them frequently. Arriving home safely is of paramount importance for both you and your child.

If your child is being admitted to the hospital, you will be transferred to the floor when the nursing and anesthesia staff feels that your child is stable. Once on the floor, you will meet the in-patient nursing staff, support staff (such as LPNs), and the attending physician. In teaching hospitals, you will also meet the resident staff taking care of your child. Many hospitals employ full-time physicians to augment the care rendered by your surgeon. Your pediatrician may or may not have responsibility for your child's care while they are hospitalized. These are issues that should be clarified with your surgeon and primary care provider prior to surgery.

If your child will be cared for by the hospital team, they will need to obtain a detailed history from you concerning your child's health and perform an examination so they can become familiar with your child's medical condition. Please be patient with this process as it is in your child's best interest to have the entire health-care team familiar with the issues that surround your child's care.

Your child will be discharged from the hospital when your surgeon—in conjunction with the hospital team and/or your pediatrician (if involved)—feel he or she is stable enough to go home. The nursing staff will review the discharge instructions provided by your child's health-care team. Please review these and make sure you understand how to care for your child in the postoperative period.

Caring for your child at home: Following surgery, your surgeon will review which activities are prohibited in the postoperative period. Children do not have the common sense that adults have developed with experience; do not rely on your child to moderate his or her activities.

I often receive calls from parents asking if their child can go to school within a few days after surgery when I have instructed that they remain out of school for one week. While your child may appear well, they need the rest and quiet environment that home affords. It is unfair to the teaching staff at your child's school to monitor their activity when they may have 18 or more children to tend to.

School is also a place where children commonly come in contact with viral and bacterial illnesses. Developing an upper respiratory tract infection immediately after surgery will slow your child's recovery. Even if your child looks great, follow your surgeon's instructions and keep them home from school. If you must go to work, find a friend or relative to stay with your child.

Discuss with your surgeon when travel is advisable. As

I counsel my patients and their families, vacation areas are wonderful for relaxation, but you may not have access to the best health care in the event of an emergency. I know my patients well and would feel much more comfortable dealing with them personally than asking them to visit an emergency room in an area where I am unfamiliar with the physicians.

What types of activities are permissible at home? This is an issue that should be discussed with your surgeon preoperatively. It may be impossible to prevent your child from playing with their siblings, but try to limit the amount of roughhousing that occurs. Having a heart-to-heart talk with an older sibling and asking them to help you in making sure their younger brother or sister has a chance to rest may empower them to be your ally in the recovery process.

Try not to put your recovering child in a situation where they must sit on the sidelines while their friends or siblings are having fun. Do not take them to the playground or pool and expect them to sit quietly while others are being active and rambunctious. It will be stressful on both of you and will not give them the rest their body needs. If you are unsure about which activities are permitted, ask your surgeon preoperatively, review these instructions again at the time of surgery, and do call your surgeons office postoperatively with questions or concerns.

During your follow-up appointment, your surgeon will give you a progress update on your child's condition. These visits are vitally important for your surgeon to assess your child's progress toward recovery, and to ascertain that the healing process is on track. In some cases, sutures need to be removed or the dressing over the surgical site needs to be changed. Be sure to schedule these appointments preoperatively so that you and your spouse or significant other can discuss how the surgery went and the recovery time frame. Make a list of questions to bring to your postoperative visit. Remember, recovery is a process and you may not see immediate results from surgery. Your surgeon can discuss with you how your child's recovery is progressing.

Chapter 8

Chronic Illness

Dealing with chronic illness in your child

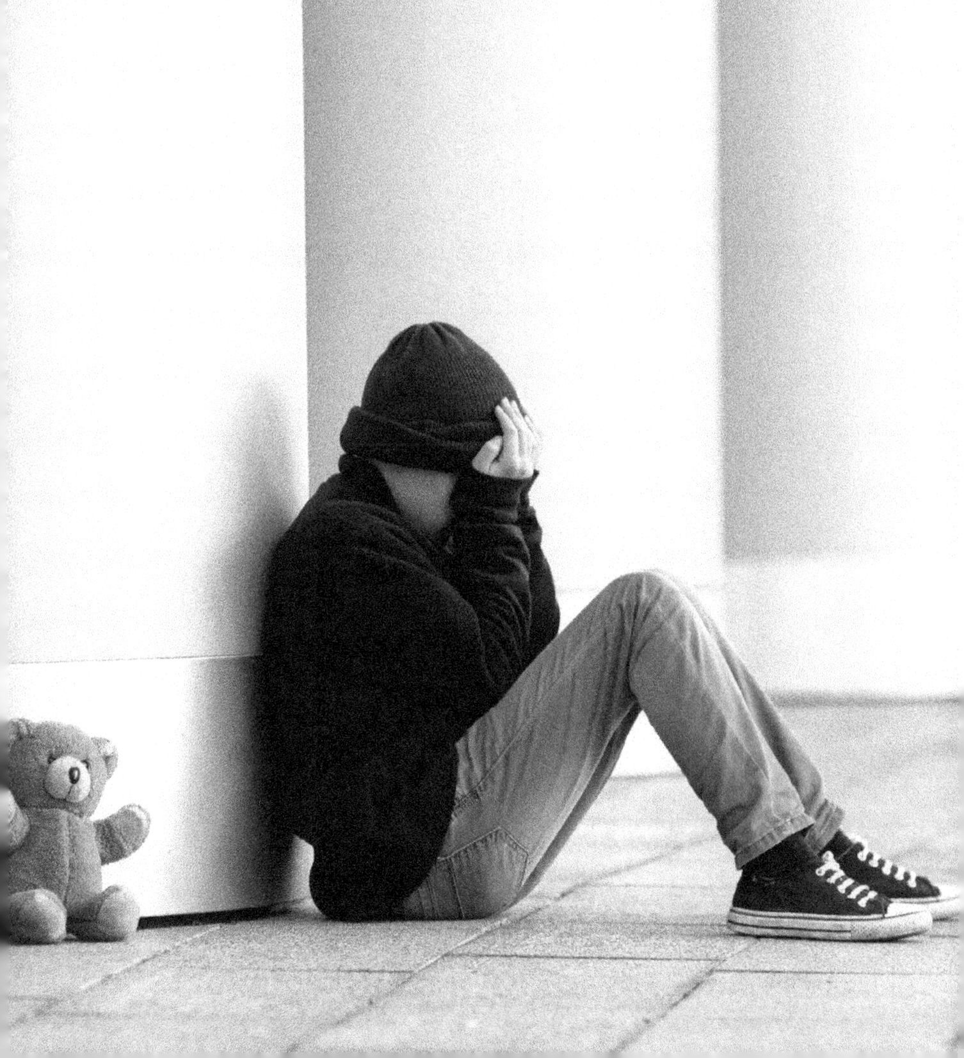

Dealing with a child with chronic illness requires a shift in our expectations as parents.

The gentle hissing of the ventilator expanding my patient's lungs greeted me as I entered the otherwise quiet room of the intensive care unit. There my young patient lay, sedated and paralyzed, keeping him from fighting the breathing machine.

I walked toward the window where his mother was sitting, wrapped in a blanket, inches from her son's bed.

"Mrs. Johnson, I'm here," I murmured, gently placing my hand on her shoulder.

Her eyes flickered open and were rimmed with the swelling of too many tears recently shed. She looked into my face with the sadness of many sleepless nights, holding her struggling child in her arms. Those nights ultimately ended in the intensive care unit each time, a breathing tube now keeping her baby alive.

Born with paralyzed vocal cords, her son had struggled for each breath since birth. His mother and I had decided we would wait as long as possible prior to placing an artificial airway in his neck to see if, as he grew, his vocal cord function would improve. He was not as lucky as others and his respiratory status worsened as he aged.

The last straw was an upper respiratory tract infection

that required hospitalization, and a breathing tube that snaked through his mouth into his lungs.

"I think it's time," she whispered.

These four simple words carried a complex message from a mother who could no longer stand to watch her child suffer.

"Of course," I reached out again to touch her shoulder. "I'll arrange for the surgery as soon as possible."

What to do when your child is diagnosed with a chronic illness: Dealing with a child with chronic illness requires a shift in our expectations as parents. Gone are the assurances that they will attend high school and college. We dare not think of marriage and grandchildren. We learn to deal with one day at a time and are grateful for the time we have with them.

It is imperative as a parent of a child with chronic illness to organize your health-care team. Who will be the primary contact person for your child's care? In most situations, this will be your primary care provider. They can help you choose your specialist and arrange for the appropriate health-care setting for your child.

The news that your child has been diagnosed with a chronic illness can be devastating. The internet should not be your primary source of information. Instead, set up a follow-up meeting, after you have had the opportunity to digest this information, and have a discussion with your child's pediatrician or primary care provider about their thoughts on your child's illness.

How serious is the condition? Are there immediate measures needed to stabilize the condition? What specialists are needed to help confirm the condition? If you have already seen a specialist, has your pediatrician had the opportunity to confer with them and develop a plan of treatment going forward?

Develop, with your pediatrician, a plan as to who will be in charge of your child's care. When issues occur, should you contact your pediatrician or the specialist?

Next, inform your child, in an age-appropriate fashion, of their diagnosis. Your pediatrician can be a great asset in helping to frame this discussion with you and your child. If your child has been hospitalized at the time the diagnosis was made, avail yourself of the child life specialist, if one is on staff. They are trained professionals who can help to support you and your child as you work through what your child's treatment will entail (e.g., X-rays, intravenous treatments, dialysis, or surgery).

Your specialist's office may also be a resource for information on your child's condition. They will have access to information which will help you to understand the changes in your life and your child's life that must occur to keep their health as stable as possible.

Building your health-care team

Primary care provider: Your pediatrician or primary care physician is, in most instances, the point person to help organize your child's care. They should be helping you to process the information about your child's diagnosis, helping you explain to your child (with their guidance and support) what their diagnosis means, and serve as a resource and support for your older children as they process this information. They can also provide medical documentation to educational agencies, your insurance company, and social services, to document the severity of your child's illness.

Make sure that all reports from your child's specialist, as well as all tests and reports from hospital admissions, are provided to your child's primary care provider's office. Keeping them informed as to the ongoing process of treatment for your child will allow them to be the best possible advocate for your child as they journey through the medical system.

Specialist: Your specialist will help develop the care plan, and will in most cases be the one you turn to and interact with primarily about recommendations for treatment. They, with your primary care provider, should be your main source of information and recommendations about treatment of your child's condition.

Make sure as you process this information that you filter, in an age-appropriate fashion, the amount of information your child receives. Work through your initial grief, anxiety, and frustration about your child's health before you and your physicians discuss the issues with your child.

If you are sobbing and inconsolable as you interact with your child about their illness, it will only raise their feelings of helplessness and despair in how to deal with their diagnosis. Most pediatric specialists are sensitive to these issues and will interact with your child in a way that will help them process the needed information with as little anxiety as possible.

Discuss with your specialist who in their office will be your primary contact.

Is there a nurse, nurse practitioner or physician's assistant who will help answer your day-to-day questions? Are there information sessions in the office or at the hospital to help educate you and your older child about their illness? Can you interact with the physician and staff via email? What do you do if an emergency occurs? What coverage is available if the physician is unavailable and what hospital or emergency room do they recommend you go to if an emergency occurs? What will be the frequency of appointments and can relatives, friends, or nannies bring your child to routine appointments if you are unavailable? Are there special forms that need to be filled out to allow others to bring your child to appointments? Will the specialist send you a written note, call you, or email you about the results of your child's visit if you do not accompany them?

What type of information from you is helpful for your specialist to have in assessing how successful their treatment protocol has been? Would they like daily logs, weekly logs, or just an overall impression? If logs would be helpful, do they have preprinted forms that are available so that you, and your child if possible, can provide information that will be useful in fine-tuning their care?

The relationship that you are entering into with your specialist will most likely be long term. Evaluate if this is a person you feel will be there for you and your child for years to come. Evaluate them from a medical standpoint, a personality standpoint, and how user-friendly the office is. If you have a teenager, it is helpful when they like their doctor as well. Remember, they may be going through a tough phase adjusting to their illness and may not like any physician, so be patient and supportive.

Though it may seem like an odd request, inquire if your specialist has any plans of moving their practice or leaving the hospital setting that would cause a change in the physician responsible for your child's care. Take the first several months to adjust to your child's specialist and be vocal about what is working and what is not.

Psychological support: The diagnosis of a chronic illness in your child will undoubtedly elicit feelings of anger, frustration, guilt and hopelessness in both you and your child. Dealing with these feelings will make you more emotionally available for your child.

What type of support do you need? Are you the type who would benefit from a disease-specific support group?

These can be wonderful sources of information from people who may be farther down the path of dealing with this process than you are. What has worked and not worked? What are the side effects you might expect with certain medications? How to deal with the emotions your child is feeling? How to ask appropriate and helpful questions of your physicians?

Support groups are a great place to unload your feelings surrounding your child's illness. These parents have experienced every emotion you have and perhaps even more if they have been dealing with this process for years. A support group is a safe place to vent, cry, and get support. I encourage every parent to at least attend a few sessions to see if they find the information and support helpful.

Discuss with your pediatrician, specialist, and your child's teachers if psychological support would be helpful for your child. Studies have shown that what we as parents worry about may not be the same concerns our children may have. Research on anxiety in children with cancer found that they worried more about not being able to engage in their usual activities than the fear of treatment or death.[6] So be attuned to their concerns and try not to displace your concerns onto them.

If you are experiencing increasing anxiety and/or depression, consider professional help. There is no stigma in admitting you need help and getting it. Chronic illness in a child can be a huge stressor to a marriage. Decide what type of mental health provider is right for you. Licensed clinical social workers and psychologists provide therapy. Psychiatrists provide medication, and in many cases therapy as well. The American Psychological Association, the Psychology Today website, the American Psychiatric Association, as well as your local hospital physician referral service, are all options for finding a talented mental health professional to fit your needs.

Spend time talking to your spouse/significant other about how the two of you can deal with the stressors that lie ahead. It is vitally important for your mental health, as well as your child's physical and mental health, that both of you are on the same page as far as treatment options and how to interact with your child and their physicians. Decide who will try to attend appointments, who will call physicians, and how you will deal with "routine parenting at home." If you feel like the stress of your child's chronic illness is having negative effects on your marriage, seek professional help. A family therapist can help your family navigate the landmines that lie ahead.

Do not forget your other children. Help them to understand, in an age-appropriate fashion, the struggles their brother or sister may be having with their health. Though it may seem tempting, do not use your other children as sounding boards for your fears. They should not know significantly more information than what you are sharing with your sick child. No matter how mature they may seem, the burden of keeping a secret or helping you deal with your anxiety or fear is too much responsibility to place on any child.

Remember to take time for yourself. Find stress-relieving activities that you can do with your spouse, significant other, or a friend. Getting your mind off your child's illness and trying to enjoy life in whatever capacity you can, will make you a better parent. Keeping yourself as physically and emotionally healthy as possible can only help your child better deal with their illness.

School professional: Your child's illness will affect their attendance at school. It is imperative that you reach out to your child's school as soon as possible after the diagnosis has been made. If your child has been chronically ill, it is likely they are aware there is a problem, but sitting down with an educational professional will help the school to plan appropriately for your child. You should be meeting with your child's teacher, the principal, and in some situations, the board of education.

Initially speak to your specialist and primary care provider about what limitations your child will have in attending school. Will there be limitations in physical activity, and will their diagnosis or treatment affect their intellectual ability?

If your child attends a private or parochial school, you must decide if the services it can provide will meet your child's long-term needs. Does the school have the resources to provide specialized transportation, aides in the classroom, and accommodations to meet your child's physical and—in some cases—emotional and cognitive limitations? Public schools are required by law to provide a wide range of services to children with chronic illness under the Individuals with Disabilities Education Act. Discuss with your child's private or parochial school if resources can be made available to adjust to your child's needs. If possible, work with your child's school: the less disruption early in their illness, the better to allow your child the opportunity to adjust to the emotional and physical changes they undoubtedly are experiencing.

Discuss with your child's educational professionals if he or she is a candidate for an Individualized Educational Program (IEP). Your child's school and school district can help structure a course of education, specific to your child and the challenges they might encounter being away from school for illness or treatment.

Your child may also require a 504 plan. This lists the physical accommodations your child will need in light of the limitations they may encounter due to their illness. This could include special transportation to and from school, accommodations in the classroom, accommodations to access the bathroom, an aide in the classroom, and accommodations to navigate school grounds.

If your child will be required to spend prolonged periods in the hospital, inquire if your child can receive a hospital-based education. These programs are staffed with qualified teachers who will work with your child's teachers and school system to assure that he or she stays as current as possible in their studies. These classes can be bedside or in a group setting in a hospital classroom. These teachers will consult with your child's medical team to decide on the best options for continuing their education while they are hospitalized. Rely on them and your medical team to set reasonable expectations about what your child has the energy to undertake while they are hospitalized.

Remember, insurance companies are large businesses and will work hard to make their services cost efficient and profitable. If there are any rules that you neglect to follow, there is a high chance that coverage for that service will be denied or reduced. As a business, they do need to be responsive to their consumers. As an individual, you have little influence; however, if you work for a large company there is a better chance your voice will be heard.

Call your human resources department and schedule an appointment. Meet with a representative and explain your child's health challenges. Ask if they can be advocates for you and your child in negotiating with the insurance company. Develop a relationship with them so you can depend on them to act in your behalf. If they are helpful, be sure and let those in positions of authority in your company know how beneficial their involvement has been.

If you are self-employed or if you purchased your insurance on your own, all hope is not lost. Reach out to your insurance agent to pressure the insurance company to provide the maximum benefits available under your plan. The more pressure the insurance company receives from its consumers, the higher the chance is that your interactions with them will be less stressful. If all else fails, resorting to legal representation may be worthwhile. Specialized health-care attorneys can help interpret if the insurance company has not lived up to the contract entered into with you and your company. You must weigh the cost of the legal fees compared to your medical bills. With a child with chronic illness, it is likely that your medical bills will far exceed how much you would be required to pay an attorney. Be sure and be clear with your attorney what your budget is for legal services, and have them keep you informed on how much work they are doing on your behalf.

Discuss your child's rights under the Americans with Disabilities Act with your lawyer. If you proceed with paperwork to declare your child to be disabled, they may qualify for government-sponsored health insurance, educational services, and/or disability payments.

Home care vs. specialized residential care: Each of us would like to have our child cared for at home, of course. You must evaluate if this is best for you and your family. In some instances, home care is extremely difficult to arrange. If your child requires a ventilator, a machine to help them breathe, or continuous intravenous fluids or medication, then specialized equipment and personnel will be required. This may or may not be covered by your insurance company, and you must consider whether your home is the place for your child to receive the highest level of care.

If you do choose to place your child in a residential facility, be sure to work with your hospital's social work department to choose a facility that is right for you and your child. If you work full-time or have other children, a facility far from your home will leave you torn between visiting your child and the other responsibilities of life. If possible, choose a facility that is dedicated to the care of children with chronic illnesses. Discuss with your insurance carrier as well as your social work team what services can be provided at home and in what situations residential care is required. Remember, no decision is set in stone, and you can change your place of care as your child's illness evolves.

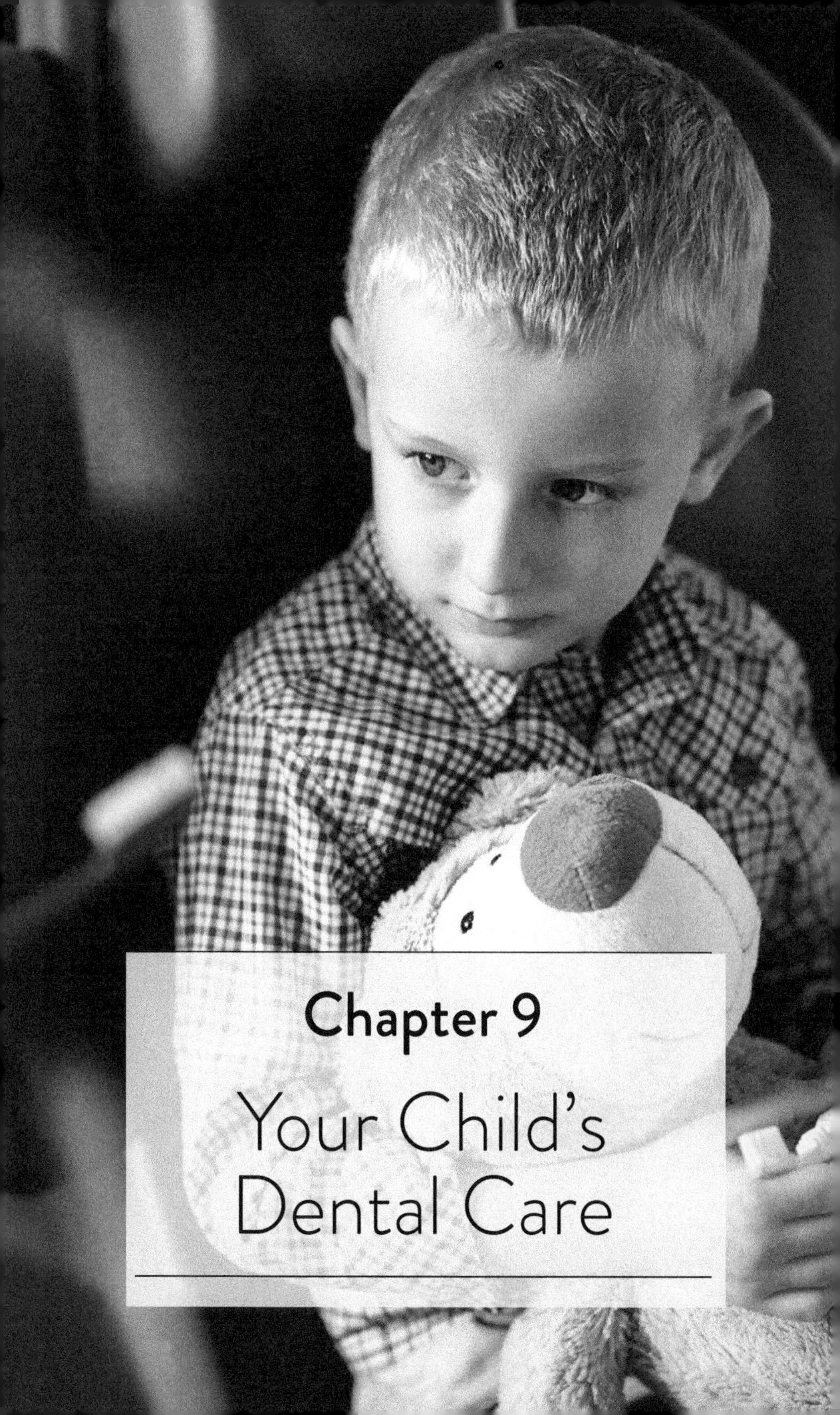

Chapter 9
Your Child's Dental Care

Children are dependent on parents
to maintain their oral health,
and as many of us know,
this can be a daily struggle.

The persistent shrill ring of the telephone penetrated my slumber. My eyes flew open and I grabbed for the phone before it awakened my husband. From years of sleeping next to me as I responded to the emergencies of my medical career, he had developed the ability to sleep through most intrusions.

I cleared the sleep from my voice as I murmured into the phone, "Dr Jones, may I help you?" My stomach sank as I heard the voice of the senior resident at the large metropolitan hospital where I worked. Arjun had joined our residency program after completing a residency in India. He was skilled, confident, and rarely called for assistance. "Sorry to wake you, Dr. Jones, but we have a pretty sick kid here in the emergency room and I think we need to go to the operating room immediately."

In succinct terms he described the case. Kayla, a six-year-old girl, had been transferred from our affiliate hospital in Queens with a severe infection in her mouth. She came from an immigrant family who had moved to the United States just a year ago. Over the past several days she had developed pain, fever and swelling in her face and neck. She had been unable to open her mouth due to the swelling and pain and a CAT scan had revealed a large collection of pus that was constricting her airway.

"I'm on my way, get the operating room ready," I barked into the phone, and I hurried to pull on my clothes.

As I entered the emergency room, the orderly chaos that surrounds a critically ill child assailed my senses. The persistent beep of the cardiac monitor, the hissing of the oxygen machine, the acrid smell of fear that emanated from the huddled bodies of her parents who stood at the foot of her bed trying to calm their terrified child, engulfed me. I performed a quick examination and tried, through a waiting translator, to explain to her parents how we would attempt to save their child. Kayla's mother grabbed my hand and began to sob uncontrollably. I squeezed her hand and turned to ensure Arjun was ready to transport the child to the operating room. Always prepared, he was already slowly moving Kayla to a bed to begin our ascent to the operating room three floors above.The next hour pushed all of us to work as a team to secure Kayla's airway and stabilize her breathing. An incision in her neck allowed the trapped infection to drain. As the tense swelling dissipated from her neck, I opened her mouth and was met with the pungent smell of rotting teeth. Well meaning and perhaps indulgent, her parents had most likely allowed Kayla to fall asleep with the sugar from a juice or milk bottle, slowly dissolving the susceptible enamel of her baby teeth. Jagged and rotting, they were most likely the source of her infection.

Oral health and your child: While the eyes may be the windows to the soul, the mouth is the window to our general health. Children are dependent on parents to maintain their oral health, and as many of us know, this can be a daily struggle. The process of enamel formation starts 15 weeks after conception and continues until 9 months after birth.[7] The enamel-producing cells are called ameloblast and are extremely sensitive to nutritional disturbances during pregnancy. The American Dental Association advises that pregnant mothers eat a variety of healthy foods including grains, fruit, and dairy products, and limit their ingestion of sugar and sugar-containing drinks. (Fig. 2).

A child's primary teeth are present at birth in the jaw and begin their eruption between 6 and 12 months of life. (Fig. 3). The first teeth to appear are the front teeth in the lower than upper jaw. It is crucial early in life to think about and prevent tooth decay. It is estimated that 75% of weak enamel in children is caused by developmental issues which can be due to prematurity, nutritional deficiency in the mother's diet, poor nutrition in early childhood, or illness in the mother during pregnancy, as well as infections in childhood. Approximately 25% of enamel deficits are due to trauma to the teeth during early childhood that can result in decreased thickness of the tooth enamel.

Dental disease is a common problem in children, with one in four children having a cavity by the time they enter kindergarten. Early recognition and treatment of dental disease can prevent tooth loss, dental infections, and the possibility of complications from untreated dental infections. A dentist should examine children during their first year of life. This is an important opportunity to develop a long-term relationship with a dentist for your child.

Choosing a dentist:

- Start your search by discussing recommendations for a dentist with your child's pediatrician or primary physician. Your child's health-care provider can direct you to a practice that has experience in treating infants and young children. The decision of choosing a pediatric dentist versus a general dentist may be based on availability of a pediatric dentist in your area.
- The internet is a never-ending source of information; use it to narrow your choices. With small children, a dentist in your neighborhood may be preferable to having to travel for routine appointments. If a health-care provider who accepts your insurance is important, visit your insurance company's website to find a list of providers. Community blogs may also be a resource for a referral to a qualified dentist.
- Your family and friends are additional sources of referrals to a good dentist. Speak to a person whose views on medical care mirror your own.
- Schedule an appointment to meet potential dentists to see if there is a fit between your personality and theirs. Meet the staff and hygienist to see if they appear friendly and outgoing.
- Assure that the dental office is child-friendly. Many dental offices have television sets in the dental exam rooms, and are brightly colored to make them visually appeal-

ing for children.

What to expect at your child's dental visits: Developing a relationship with a caring professional dentist is the first step in assuring your child's optimum dental health. Schedule the visit when you feel your child will be at their best and well rested. For toddler and older children, perhaps consider choosing a special "visit the dentist outfit" to make it a special occasion.

Make sure your child eats prior to their exam so they will not be hungry or cranky. Clean your child's teeth so they are not caked with food. Try and be relaxed and positive about the exam. Your child will be sensitive to your mood and will be calmer about the exam if you are.

Go online and fill out the registration form prior to the visit to ensure you can concentrate on your child in the waiting room and keep them as relaxed and positive as possible.

During your child's first dental visit, they will sit on your lap in a comfortable roomy chair. The dentist will examine the structures of the mouth and check that your child's teeth are erupting in a normal manner. They will make sure no cavities are developing and will, as your child ages, clean their teeth periodically. During these initial visits, your child's dentist will discuss how to clean your baby's mouth as well as how to effectively brush your child's emerging teeth and use fluorinated toothpaste in a safe and effective manner.

Raise any concerns you may have about teething, pacifier use, and thumb sucking during these routine visits.

Your child should be seen by a dentist every six months. Expect the first set of X-rays at four to six years of age, to check for cavities lurking deep in the tooth. Children will routinely need dental X-rays every five years unless a problem develops. You have every right as a parent to discuss the use of X-rays for your child. The vast majority of dental offices adhere to the "image gently campaign." These recommendations by the American College of Radiology suggest that the minimal amount of radiation needed to perform a study should be used. It is not a single X-ray that increases a child's risk of cancer, but the cumulative effect of radiation over their life span.

Having an open discussion with your dentist about how frequently X-rays are required, and about using the lowest dose of radiation possible, will assure your child receives quality care with minimal exposure.

Prevention of dental cavities in children: Your child's health-care providers will review the importance of good nutrition on your child's health. Poor nutrition can have profound effects on the strength of your child's teeth and the tendency to develop cavities early in life.

Breastfeeding is the best source of nutrition in infancy. The World Health Organization recommends that mothers exclusively breastfeed their children for the first six months of life. Research has shown that children who breastfeed during the first year of life have a lower incidence of dental cavities than children who were formula fed.[9] A 2017 study in the journal *Pediatrics* has reported a 2.4% higher incidence of severe cavities in children who are breastfed for more than two years of life. In children who are breastfed past 24 months, strict adherence to good oral hygiene is recommended.[10]

Cavity-causing bacteria can be passed to your newborn via your saliva. Prior to eruption of your child's first tooth, their mouth is free of cavity-forming bacteria. For cavities to form, three factors must be present: teeth, sugar, and cavity-forming bacteria. The most common source of cavity-forming bacteria is saliva from a parent or caregiver.[11] Babies are most susceptible to being infected with cavity-forming bacteria during the first nine months of life when the tooth enamel is hardening. Kissing your infant on the mouth, licking their utensils or pacifier are common avenues for the introduction of cavity-forming bacteria to infants. Avoid passing saliva to your child and thoroughly clean all utensils, pacifiers, and toys that enter their mouth.

Avoid the introduction of increased sugar to your child's diet. It is impossible and somewhat cruel to completely avoid sugar but limit their exposure to sugar-based drinks and food. Make sugar-containing foods and drink an infrequent special treat.

Parents should avoid putting children to sleep with a bottle where milk or sugar-containing products have the potential for prolonged exposure to developing teeth. Limiting sugar exposure will increase the chances of optimal dental health for your child.

Orthodontic care for your child: When is the appropriate time to have your child evaluated by an orthodontist? Your pediatric dentist will be the best guide as to when your child needs an orthodontic evaluation. The American Association of Orthodontists suggests that children be evaluated at approximately seven years of age. Early evaluation of your child can prevent the development of facial bone deformities due to dental misalignment. Warning signs to suggest your child should see an orthodontist include:

- Chronic mouth breathing
- Excessive teeth grinding
- An obvious overbite or underbite
- Teeth that are crowded or not aligned
- Thumb sucking that persists after four years of age

Children who are chronic mouth breathers run the risk of poor alignment of the teeth, as well as the risk of improper development of the upper jaw and bones of the roof of the mouth or hard palate. The facets in our teeth help the upper and lower teeth align and stay in the correct position. If your child is chronically mouth breathing, the teeth have a greater opportunity to shift as your child grows. Having your child breath through their nose and having their mouth closed helps the upper jaw to grow correctly. Without pressure from the teeth and lower jaw, the upper jaw or maxilla will continue to grow and will result in an abnormally long face. This excess growth of the maxilla can also affect the bone at the roof of the mouth and contribute to abnormal development of these bones. Chronic mouth breathing can be caused by blockage of the nose. Your pediatric dentist or orthodontist in consultation with your child's pediatrician, and if needed an ear, nose and throat specialist, can help to ascertain the cause and best treatment to alleviate chronic mouth breathing.

Many children grind their teeth. The most common ages for teeth grinding are when the baby teeth begin to emerge and when the permanent teeth erupt. Most teeth grinding is self-limited and will resolve. Concern arises if teeth grinding become excessive and the facets of the teeth are ground away. If left untreated, this can lead to teeth misalignment, and in older children, damage to permanent teeth.[12]

Teeth grinding in children can be caused by various factors, such as misalignment of the teeth or jaw, emotional issues such as stress or anxiety, or tooth pain. A thorough evaluation of your child's teeth by a trained pediatric dentist is recommended for any child with excessive teeth grinding.

An obvious overbite or underbite are signs that your child's teeth and jaw are not developing in optimum aligment for good dental health. The earlier these issues are identified and addressed, the sooner they can be corrected.

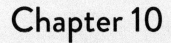

Chapter 10
Nutrition

Maximizing nutrition for your child

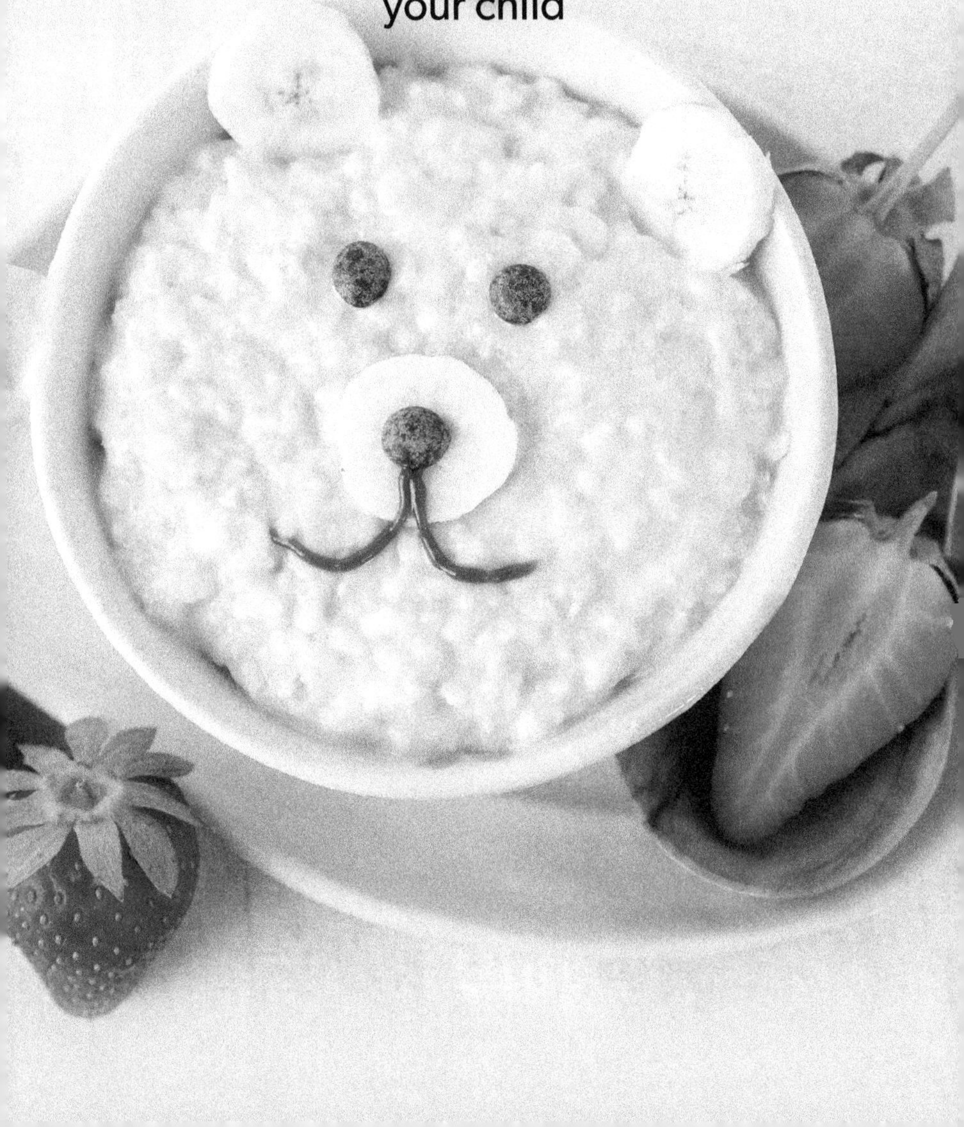

Research has shown that brain development is dependent on adequate nutrients being provided to the developing brain.

I perched over my desk finishing up the last few charts of the day. Both my boys were home from school and I was relishing the opportunity to spend time with them at the family dinner table. I had stayed up late making their favorite meal, lasagna with homemade sauce. The recipe had been passed down from my grandmother and had the extra ingredient of chili powder in the sauce to give it that southern heat she had so dearly loved. My boys always came back for second and third helpings. I had prepared a Caesar salad and warm garlic bread to complete the meal. I figured I had them captured for at least 30-40 minutes of family time before the lure of friends and video games stole them from my grasp.

"Dr. Jones, so sorry but there is one more patient I really need you to see." I looked up to see the worried face of Rachel, my medical assistant, looking down upon me.

"This Mom called a short while ago and she is really worried about her one year old son. She says he just can't stop coughing and the urgent care center keeps telling her it's a cold." Rachel had been with us for several years and I had watched her grow from an inexperienced young girl to a confident young women who worked all day and was attending school at night to earn her RN. She was smart and dedicated and I trusted her clinical judgment, she was usually right.

“No problem Rachel, I’ll be right in. “

As I walked down the hall a constant barking cough emanated from my exam room. As I entered the room I watched as this small one-year boy played with his mothers phone while he incessantly coughed with every few breaths.

“Thank you so much for waiting for me. It’s a pleasure to meet you. Please tell me a little bit about what’s been going on with your beautiful boy” I smiled at his mother trying to put her somewhat at ease

She smiled back. Happy, I assumed, to see a smiling face. “ Doctor thank you so much for seeing us. I’m so frustrated. Drew has been coughing for two weeks and nothing seems to be helping. I have been to the urgent care center twice and he has been on nebulizers with no improvement”

I spent the next twenty minutes listening to Drew’s history and examining him. When I listened to his lungs there was a wheeze on the right side that was pronounced. I asked a few more in-depth questions and the cause of Drew cough became more apparent.

“Do you remember anything special that might have occurred two weeks ago? Was Drew with a new babysitter or at a friend’s house with you? “ I inquired.

“As a matter of fact I did take Drew to my friends house with his older brother. She was having a few friends over and I thought it would be a nice break. Oh no, you don’t think he could have gotten into something do you? “ Fear swept across her face.

“I’m a little concerned about that. Let’s send him over to

the hospital for an x-ray and make sure."

The call came as I walked in the front door of my apartment, the smell of lasagna and garlic bread wafting through the air.

I punched the number to the emergency room into my phone and received the news I expected to hear. Drew's x-ray showed an object lodged in the breathing passage that supplied air to his right lung. I sighed and turned to head back out the door as the boys and my husband gathered at the dinner table.

The surgery went well and the fragments of peanut were successfully removed from Drew's breathing passages and his lung began to expand immediately.

I sat with Mom as she cried while her baby slept peacefully for the first time in over two weeks.

"I feel so terrible. I asked his older brother about the party and he said he gave Drew a few peanuts to eat. He said Drew just grabbed them and he thought he might like them so he gave him a few more. I can't believe how stupid he was. Look what's happened. I'm a horrible mother!" The tears rolled down her cheeks as her sobbing intensified.

"Please don't beat up on yourself or your older son. It was an accident and I'm sure it won't happen again. The important thing is he is fine now and you will recover in time as well. Just not as quickly." I squeezed her hand. " I'll be back in the morning. Don't worry he is doing well and hopefully you will be going home tomorrow."

A pile of dirty dishes awaited me as I entered my kitchen, but off to the corner was a plate of lasagna, salad and bread with a glass of wine next to it. I grabbed my meal and headed to my son's room where the sound of video games, laughing and male bonding emanated as the boys endeavored to teach their father the intricacies of their latest game. I settled onto the floor as I watched another alien bite the dust as the roar of gunfire exploded from the big screen TV. I would take my quality time with my boys where ever and whenever I could get it.

As mothers, we have all experienced the frustration of trying to get our children, whether they be toddlers or teenagers, to eat a healthy diet. The frustration is that as parents we know the importance of good nutrition through all stages of development. Research has shown that brain development is dependent on adequate nutrients being provided to the developing brain. The best source of vitamins and minerals is from whole foods.

Birth to six months: Breastfeeding has been demonstrated to be the best source of nutrition for the newborn. Nutritious breast milk is dependent on a well-rounded diet in the mother. Adequate intake of iron, folate and vitamins is necessary to provide quality breast milk. During pregnancy and lactation, the body responds to the increased caloric needs by increasing appetite.

Women are usually advised to increase their caloric intake by 20%–25% to meet the additional demands of pregnancy and lactation. Increased caloric intake does not routinely affect the amount of breast milk produced. This is dependent on how often and how vigorously the baby feeds.

Increased frequency of breastfeeding leads to increased production of breast milk. Your baby's weight will be followed carefully during the first few months of life to assure they are obtaining adequate nutrition. In some cases, your pediatrician may weigh your child before and after breastfeeding to assess how much milk they consume during an average feed.

If you are having problems with breastfeeding, consult your pediatrician early. It is common in first-time mothers to struggle the first few weeks after delivery with breastfeeding. Meeting with a lactation consultant will be useful in helping both you and your pediatrician understand why you might be struggling. Most hospitals have lactation consultants on staff to provide consultations prior to your discharge. A lactation consultant is an allied health professional who is trained to teach mothers how to feed their infants. Lactation consultants require a minimum of 90 hours of lactation education. They can receive certification through the International Board of Lactation Consultants after completing 1,000 hours of supervised clinical experience with breastfeeding mothers and their infants. A lactation consultant will examine both the mother's breast as well as the baby's oral cavity. They are looking for problems with the mother's breast such as inverted or retracted nipples, prior breast surgery, or infection. The lactation consultant will examine your child's mouth and lips to evaluate if their tongue or lips are restricted by extra skin (a tongue or lip tie), if they have adequate strength to produce an effective suck or if there are any anatomic problems with the jaw, tongue, or soft tissues inside the mouth that could interfere with breastfeeding. A lactation consultant, as well as your child's primary care provider, will work with you to maximize your child's ability to breastfeed.

Most children tolerate breast milk without issues. However, frequent spitting up or reflux may be a sign of breast milk or formula intolerance.

I advise parents to watch for spitting up of a tablespoon or more at the majority of feedings as this may be a warning sign of gastroesophageal reflux. All babies experience some gastroesphageal reflux—that is, the passing of stomach contents up the feeding tube (esophagus) into the mouth. This is due to lower tone in the muscle, which separates the stomach from the esophagus in infants. This tone improves as the baby matures. Gastroesophageal reflux can result in a small amount of spitting up or significant vomiting depending upon the severity. Severe reflux, if left untreated, can result in malnutrition and weight loss. Reflux can present at any time during the first six months of life, and in most children improves with the introduction of solid food at approximately six months of age. Reflux can be the result of milk protein allergies in some children and if your child is spitting up at the majority of feeds, they should be evaluated by their pediatrician

Milk protein allergy is the most common allergy in children. In newborns, milk protein is passed from breast milk to the infant during breastfeeding. A true allergy is different from intolerance. Allergies are immune mediated and typically present with more severe symptoms than in those children with intolerance to foods. Milk protein allergy is much less common in children who are exclusively breastfed as compared to children who receive formula exclusively or receive supplemental formula. Food intolerance is uncommon in children less than two years of age. Common symptoms of milk protein allergy in infants are diarrhea that can be severe and bloody. Additional symptoms which can be present, depending upon the severity of the allergy, are wheezing, difficulty breathing, nasal congestion and vomiting. It is estimated that 50%–60% of children with milk protein allergy will have skin reactions such as dermatitis and 50%–60% of children will manifest gastrointestinal symptoms such as reflux, diarrhea, or vomiting. Approximately 20%–30% will present with respiratory symptoms such as runny nose, cough, sneezing and an increased number of ear infections.[13]

Your child's physician can best diagnoses a milk protein allergy. They will perform a thorough history and physical examination. They will ask about your family history of allergies. If one parent has allergies, there is an approximate 30% chance of their offspring having allergies. If both parents have allergies, there is an approximate 60% chance of their children having allergies. After completion of the history and physical exam, your health care provider may do additional testing. They will commonly examine your child's stool for the presence of blood which is a warning sign of cow's milk allergy. If the history and physical exam are suggestive of a mild to moderate cow's milk allergy, an elimination diet will be suggested. If your child has severe symptoms of allergies, such as swelling of the lips or tongue, difficulty breathing, or severe vomiting causing weight loss, referral to an allergist, who may perform blood or skin tests, will most likely be recommended.

In an elimination diet, in an exclusively breastfed child, cow's milk as well as hen's eggs are eliminated from the mother's diet. Hen's egg allergy is the second most common cause of allergies in infants and young children, after cow's milk protein allergies. Therefore, in babies with evidence of food allergies, hen's eggs should be removed from the mother's diet. Peanut protein is also passed through breast milk and has the potential to produce life-threatening allergies in children. There is concern that early exposure to peanuts in allergic children may lead to sensitization later in childhood; therefore, peanuts should also be avoided in the mother's diet. Your pediatrician will usually recommend a minimum of 2–4 weeks on an elimination diet to see if your child's symptoms improve. If there is improvement, your health care provider will recommend, as your child ages, to slowly add in one food per week to your diet to see if the introduction of new foods affects your child's symptoms. A breastfeeding mother on an elimination diet should consult her physician on the need for calcium supplementation to her diet.

In formula fed infants who are diagnosed with milk protein allergy, a change in formula is indicated. It is estimated that approximately 10% of children with milk protein allergies will be allergic to soy. Therefore, in children with cow's milk protein allergy, a soy-based formula should be avoided.

Most pediatricians recommend extensively hydrolyzed formulas (eHF). These formulas are hypoallergenic and "predigested." In an eHF the milk protein (casein) is broken down and is much easier for the infant's GI tract to absorb. Examples of eHF are Alimentum® and Nutramigen®. If your child is unable to tolerate an extensively hydrolyzed formula, your pediatrician may suggest an amino acid-based formula (AAF). These formulas are made from 100% amino acids that decease the chance of your child developing allergies. Examples of AAF are Neocate® and EleCare®. These formulas can be more expensive than other formulas, so you should discuss with your pediatrician and your insurance company options for reimbursement if your child will require long-term use of an AAF. Most allergies in children will resolve as they age and it is unlikely that your child's milk protein allergy will continue into early childhood.

Six months to two years old: As your infant reaches the six-month mark, your pediatrician or primary care provider will recommend the introduction of food to your child's diet. This is an exciting time for both you and your child as they transition to participating in mealtime with your family. The first foods to be introduced are either rice or oatmeal cereal. These are usually introduced between five to six months of age. Rice and oats are easily digested and can be mixed with breast milk or formula to a porridge consistency. You can start with one tablespoon of this cereal one to three times per day, and slowly increase the amount as your baby matures. Use a soft-tipped baby spoon to avoid irritating your baby lips and gums when feeding.

Both rice and oatmeal can be constipating. If your child is experiencing constipation, discuss with your pediatrician if the introduction of prunes, apples, or pears or adding more water to their diet would be beneficial.

Other foods that can be introduced to an infant's diet at six months of age include pureed vegetables such as sweet potatoes and squash, as well as pureed fruits such as apples, pears, bananas, and peaches. If possible, prepare your child's food from fresh, organic fruits and vegetables. Be sure to wash all fruits and vegetables thoroughly before cooking.If you use food from a jar, transfer the contents to a bowl to avoid contaminating the jar with bacteria from either your mouth or your child's mouth. Begin with a small amount of fruits or vegetables (one teaspoon) one to three times per day, and slowly increase this amount over the next several weeks. Introduce one food at a time and wait at least three days before introducing another food. Record any reaction your baby may have to a new food and avoid retrying that food until you discuss the reaction with your child's health care provider.

Food aversion is common in infants. It may take several tries to get your child to feel comfortable eating from a spoon and accepting new tastes and consistencies of food. Be sure to have the majority of their calories obtained from either breast milk or formula during this transition stage. Your pediatrician will help develop a feeding schedule with you during the slow process of transitioning to solid food. Allow your child to be an adventurous eater. Just because you hate squash does not mean your child will hate it as well. Conversely, just as you love sweet potatoes your child may hate them from birth. Never force a particular food as your child may be telling you their body cannot process that food or may even be allergic to it. Try again in one week and if they have the same reaction, avoid that food for several months. Consider adding meat stews, fish and whole grains which are well cooked and pureed to your child's diet. Spicy foods and sour foods are fed to babies throughout the world, so be adventurous and slowly expand your child's diet.

Your baby's body is not yet able to digest whole milk and you should avoid introducing whole milk until they are one year of age. Avoid putting your child to sleep with a bottle in their mouth, especially a bottle filled with sugar-containing liquids such as juice, formula, or breast milk. Feed your baby and then help them transition to bedtime without the crutch of a sugary bottle that can promote serious tooth decay.

As your child ages, you will be introducing more solid food to their diet. As soon as your baby is comfortably able to sit up, position a high chair at the dining table. Children model what they are exposed to.

If your child sees his parent and siblings eating in a relaxed environment, mealtime becomes an enjoyable time for them and they are more quickly integrated into the family structure. All of our lives are busy, and it may be inconvenient to have your baby wait until 7p.m. or 8 p.m. when the rest of the family is eating. Try to include your infant whenever possible and make the meals you have together as a family enjoyable and stress-free.

As your child reaches one year of age, more of their nutrition will be coming from solid food as compared to breast milk or formula. If approved by your pediatrician, you can start to introduce whole milk at one year of age. Young children need the fats and nutrients in whole milk and you should avoid low fat or skim milk until after two years of age.

Most pediatricians recommend limiting milk, formula, or breast milk intake to 16 ounces per day as long as your child has a diet containing iron-rich foods like fish, beans, meat, and vegetables. They should continue to eat iron-fortified cereal until two years of age. Baby-led weaning is a process where you give your child larger pieces of soft foods to allow them to transition to a more solid diet. This can begin when your baby is able to tolerate pureed foods, and this form of feeding should be discussed with your child's primary care provider.

Teaching self-feeding is an important transition for both you and your child. The less time you spend trying to "shovel" food into your baby's mouth, the more time you can "attempt to relax" and enjoy your mealtime with your family and child. At approximately 7–8 months of age, your child will begin grabbing for food. At approximately 9–10 months of age, they will use multiple fingers to pick up foods. Start each feeding session by holding a piece of food in your fingers and allow them to grab the item from your hands. Be patient with your child and allow them the opportunity to practice their skills and not become frustrated. As your child becomes more proficient with feeding, introduce a spoon. Allow your child to hold the spoon in their hand and help them dip the spoon in food and move it towards their mouth. By two years of age, the vast majority of children will have mastered self-feeding.

As your child transitions to a more solid diet, be mindful that they do not have the oro-motor coordination that an older child will have. They will be more likely to choke on foods than an older child.

Two to four years old: Until four years of age, your child will have difficulty chewing and swallowing certain foods. This is in part due to their erupting teeth, poor oro-motor coordination, and their lack of concentration during mealtime. As a parent, it is our responsibility to ensure nutritious, safe foods for our children. Foods that should be very closely monitored during mealtime or snack time (or avoided) are popcorn, whole grapes, cherries, and even blueberries in young children. Sticky foods such as peanut butter, gum, caramels, dried fruit, and fruit leathers should be monitored or avoided. Raw vegetables such as carrots, as well as nuts and hot dogs, should be avoided as well. If your child chokes on them, hot dogs have one of the highest potentials to cause death. This is because the skin of the hot dog allows it to stay in a large chunk and block your child's breathing passages. Until four years of age, remove the skin from hot dogs and monitor your child's eating closely. Supervise mealtime in young children and avoid roughhousing at the table with older siblings. Mealtime should be a relaxed time for all members of the family.

Eating habits are established early in life, and this is the time to be wary of your child falling into what I term the "beige diet"—chicken nuggets, pasta, white rice, cheese sticks, yogurt, and milk. If you allow their palates to be limited early on it will be more difficult to introduce a varied diet as they age. Start early by feeding your toddler what the rest of the family is eating, either pureed or cut into age-appropriate pieces. Encourage them to be part of the family meal. One child should not be leaving the table to watch television in the next room while his siblings are still eating dinner. Respect family mealtime and leave your cell phone and computer in the other room. Concentrate on the joy of being together and sharing a meal.

Children are exceptionally smart at discovering how far they can push us before we cave into their demands. Set rules for mealtime and stick by them.

Your child will not become malnourished if they miss one or two meals. Don't turn mealtime into warfare, but encourage them to be a part of family mealtime so it will be less stressful and less work in the long run for you as a parent. If mealtime continues to be a battle, consult your child's health care provider for additional suggestions.

Your child will be maturing out of their baby fat stage from two to four years of age. The average weight gain for a three-year-old child is four to six pounds per year with an average gain in height of two to three inches per year. Your child's primary care provider will monitor your child's weight gain during their yearly visits. If your child has slow weight gain, your pediatrician will ask you to examine your child's diet. Are there too many empty calories in their diet such as would occur with juices, candy, or cookies? Is there enough protein and vegetables to provide adequate nutrients? Your pediatrician will ask you to maximize your child's intake of good quality foods, and limit sweets and foods with empty calories such as popcorn and chips. If your child is still not able to gain weight, a thorough medical evaluation will be undertaken to assure that there are no medical causes for your child's slow weight gain. In some cases, nutritional supplementation is indicated but in the vast majority of cases, a well-rounded healthy diet will help your child achieve an age appropriate weight.

If there is a family history of obesity in your family, your pediatrician will follow your child's weight gain closely. Overweight children are more likely to become overweight adults with the host of medical and social consequences that can result from obesity. Addressing your child's weight during their toddler years can have a significant impact on their future health. As in adults, weight gain occurs when we consume more energy than we use. Your pediatrician will do a complete history and physical exam, and calculate a body mass index which is a measure of body fat compared to height and weight. It is a fairly sensitive measurement in comparing if your child is overweight compared to children of his or her age.

It is rare for children to be required to go on strict calorie-cutting diets if they are found to be overweight. Your pediatrician will initially recommend a healthy balanced diet and increasing your child's physical activity. Switching to low fat milk, eliminating cookies, cakes and chocolate, and avoiding or diluting sweetened juices with water will help to eliminate empty calories. Have your child walk whenever possible instead of being strapped in a stroller. Look at local gyms and youth agencies for age-appropriate gym classes to get your toddler engaged and moving. If there is continued weight gain or if your child's BMI continues to be abnormal, your pediatrician may recommend consultation with a nutritionist and endocrinologist to help your child achieve a healthy weight.

Five years to adolescence: As school starts, the importance of teaching healthy eating habits becomes even more important. Your child will spend increasing amounts of time in the care of others and will be eating one to two meals per day outside the home. The adage that breakfast is the most important meal of the day should be taken to heart by all parents. The morning is a stressful time for the whole family with getting ready for work and school and the inevitable battle of getting your child out of bed, dressed, with their homework and sports equipment packed and out the door on time. Oh and make sure you are dressed, fed and ready for work for the day as well! Breakfast can fall by the wayside and it is our jobs as parents to ensure that does not happen. Make breakfast, if possible, a relaxed time in the morning. Spend the extra 15 minutes prior to going to bed to get cereal bowls out and filled, fruit cut up, and lunch boxes partially filled. Make a large bowl of oatmeal on

Sunday night that can last several days and can be sweetened with berries or fruit in the morning. Boil a few eggs and serve them with whole grain toast. Yogurt parfaits with fruit and granola, peanut butter and bananas, pancakes that have been made ahead of time, frozen and reheated with syrup and fruit, can all provide a nutritious varied breakfast for you and your children. Make sure that children understand that sitting down and eating breakfast in the morning is not negotiable and that continued discussion on this point will not be successful. You and your children will appreciate getting to work, school, or starting your day with a full stomach and a hopefully clear mind.

School lunch is always a challenge. School lunches have evolved since the days when I was a child, when soda and pasta were common on the menu. School lunches must now meet the standards of the School Nutrition Association that sets standard for these lunches to meet national nutritional standards. Soda is no longer offered in school lunches and the amount of sugar consumed in a school lunch is closely monitored. The National School Lunch Program ensures that lower income children can receive free lunch, and in some states breakfast at no charge. An application and eligibility requirements can be obtained at the United States Department of Agriculture website.

A movement called "Opt Out of School Lunch" is encouraging more schools to opt out of the federally managed school lunch program. This has consequences for the school district, as they no longer receive federal funding for their school lunches. The increasingly rigid standards for school lunches have made some school districts look harder at the pros and cons of being involved in the federal lunch program. Opting out of the federal program is more difficult for disadvantaged and urban schools where a higher percentage of children might receive federal assistance through the National School Lunch Program. For some parents, the ability to have more control over what their children eat at lunch is attractive. As a parent, being an active member of your school community and voicing your views will give you and your child the best chance of obtaining choices and a healthy balanced meal at lunchtime.

For working and busy parents, getting a healthy varied meal on the table night after night can be a challenge. As a working mother of two boys, I dreaded the "what … again, Mom" comments at dinner. Trying to come up with inventive meals that would suit my boys varied palates was always a challenge. To help organize myself, I would make a master calendar at the beginning of the month and record daily what I had made. I tried to set up a ten-day rotation of meals that my sons would enjoy. I tried to plan ahead by cooking several meals on the weekend and freezing them. When possible I tried to involve my boys in the process of preparing meals, even if it was as simple as setting the table and helping to clean up. The important message was that we all could contribute to the family meal. As we sat down to eat, my husband and I would talk about the high and low points of our days. Our boys would then be asked to share their high points, and if they felt like sharing, their low points. The point was that we connected and shared with each other. As your children age, find new and original ways to connect. Whether it is playing trivia games together, or discussing a recent movie you have all seen, or playing hangman—try anything that will allow your children to connect with you.

Adolescence to young adulthood: Connecting with your adolescent child is always difficult and mealtimes are no exception. If you have worked hard to establish family meals as an important part of their shared experience, they will be less likely to find excuses to skip meals with you. Encourage your adolescent to be a part of the conversation but don't force their involvement. They are processing their need for independence and I was always grateful that they joined us at the family dinner table without too much of a fight.

Eating disorders: Adolescence is a time when body image and weight are important to teenagers. It is also a time of hormonal changes and rapid weight gain. Helping your child to have a positive self-image and deal with their weight gain is crucial during this time. Our modern society puts pressure on women to be beautiful and thin. It is especially hard for teenagers as their sense of self is just developing. They are bombarded with images in the media of wafer-thin female models or the muscular lean and toned bodies of male actors and celebrities. This unrealistic body image, as well as the pressure from family and friends to achieve a more desirable body image, can lead a teenager down the destructive path of an eating disorder.

The signs of a developing eating disorder may be subtle at first. These can include:

- Excessive dieting or preoccupation with weight
- An exaggerated fear of being fat or gaining weight
- An altered negative self-image
- Binge eating or the disappearance of large quantities of food from the house at random times
- Dressing in layers to hide advancing weight loss
- Making comments about being overweight or fat
- Maintaining a rigid and at times excessive exercise program which is not effected by fatigue, illness, or injury
- Withdrawing from social interactions and becoming isolated
- Preparing food for others but not eating.
- Eating in secret
- Personality changes
- Frequent disappearance after eating

Physical signs of an eating disorder:

- Excessively dry, scaly skin
- Translucent color to the skin

- Orange hue to the skin from ingestion of large quantities of vegetables
- Brittle, thinning hair
- Cracked and brittle nails
- Bloating and distention of the abdomen
- Excessive constipation or diarrhea
- Pitting of the teeth with enamel wear from excessive vomiting
- Swelling of the hands and feet
- Mottled appearance of the hands and feet
- Lack of focus and concentration
- Dizziness
- Lethargy
- Loss of a period in menstruating females

Adapted from Warning Signs and Symptoms. National Eating Disorders Association. www.nationaleatingdisorders.org/learn/by-eating-disorder/anorexia/warning-signs-symptoms.
Accessed December 2017.

Eating disorders in teens are more common than previously reported. A 2007 study in the *Journal of Abnormal Psychology* followed 496 adolescent girls for 8 years until the age of 20. They found that 5.4% of their study population suffered from anorexia, bulimia or severe binge eating which was significant enough to meet the psychiatric criteria for an eating disorder. When they included nonspecific eating disorders, that number increased to 13.2% of their study population suffering from a significant eating disorder by 20 years of age.[14]

Binge eating: The most common eating disorder in the United States is binge eating. Binge eating is characterized by eating large quantities of food in a short amount of time, feeling a loss of the ability to control one's eating during the episode, and experiencing distress such as shame, guilt, or depression about the event. Binge eating is not associated with purging behaviors such as vomiting or excessive laxative use.

Binge eating has an average age of onset during the late teenage years to early 20s. There is a significantly higher incidence of obesity in individuals that binge eat as well as a higher incidence of depression and anxiety. Researchers have proposed that binge eating is associated with low self-esteem and an altered view of one's body image which can result in using food to counteract negative emotions.[15] Compared to other eating disorders, almost 40% of patients diagnosed with binge eating are males and almost one third of patients seeking weight loss treatment in the United States have signs of binge eating.

Signs of binge eating include three or more of the following behaviors:

- Eating more quickly than a normal individual

- Eating quantities of food until discomfort occurs
- Eating large quantities of food even when not feeling hungry
- Eating in secret due to embarrassment or distress over the quantity of food eaten
- Feeling significant shame, guilt, anxiety, or depression after an episode of binge eating

Adapted from Binge Eating Disorders. National Eating Disorders Association. www.nationaleatingdisorders.org/binge-eating-disorder. Accessed December 2017.

Parental attitudes toward food have also been found to affect how children interact with food as they age. Studies have shown that strict parental control of a child's diet may have the potential for abnormal eating patterns. In a 1998 study in *Pediatrics*, researchers showed that children whose parents imposed strict dietary control had a higher preference for high-fat and high-calorie foods. These children were also less likely to choose a variety of foods, and did not respond to bodily cues that they were hungry or full, and therefore had a tendency to have less control over their caloric intake in a 24-hour period.[16] Children need the opportunity to regulate their own diets to some degree, especially as they age. This study showed that parents who exerted strict control of multiple aspects of their child's diet such as what, when, and how much they ate, affected how their children interacted with food later in life.

Binge eating is a widespread problem affecting girls and

boys in all socioeconomic classes. Binge eating can have profound effects on young people's lives for years to come and has the potential for serious health consequences. Treatment of binge eating focuses on achieving recognition of the severity of the problem by the child or young adult, and addressing psychological and medical issues—as well as involving the family in providing a program of stepped therapy that addresses the severity of the problem.

Anorexia nervosa: Approximately 0.9% of all American women and 0.3% of all men will suffer from anorexia in their lifetime. Twenty-five percent of patients diagnosed with anorexia are males and they have been noted to have a higher risk of dying from the disease, due in part to delays in diagnosis.[17]

Anorexia nervosa is characterized by an altered self-image about one's weight. Being concerned about self-image and weight is a natural occurrence in teenagers.

As they negotiate where they stand on the social ladder and how others of the same or opposite sex view them, concerns about body image arise. Problems develop when this altered view of their self-image becomes destructive, and harmful behavior develops.

Many adolescents who go on to suffer from anorexia start with normal dieting. However as they lose weight they are unable to alter their image of themselves. This distorted body image leads to increasing efforts to become thinner and thinner. Much of their day is spent thinking about food, weight and their body image. The anorexic teen or young adult will go to extreme length to control his or her food intake and has an intense fear of being fat.

Some of the warning signs of anorexia nervosa include:

- Avoidance or refusal to eat
- Inability to acknowledge hunger, even when starving
- Lack of focus or difficulty concentrating
- Preoccupation with body size and shape
- Making excuses for not eating
- Restricting the type of foods which are eaten with the common avoidance of foods containing fat or sugar
- Preoccupation with the quantity of food eaten, excessively weighing food, and restricting the amount of food in the house or on one's plate
- Exhibiting abnormal behaviors when eating, such as moving food around the plate without eating it, cutting food into minute pieces, or spitting food out after chewing
- Purging after eating, by vomiting or the excessive use of laxatives
- Excessive weight loss with the inability to recognize the severity of the weight loss

Adapted from Anorexia Symptoms and Effects. Timberline Knolls. http://www.timberlineknolls.com/eating-disorder/anorexia/sign-effects/. Accessed December 2017.

The danger of anorexia is the profound effect it can have on the body. The National Eating Disorders Association estimates that young people between the ages of 15–24 with anorexia have a 10 times higher risk of dying from their disease as compared to other young people of their age. Researcher estimate that 5%–10% of anorexics die within 10 years of developing the disease, and as many as 20% will die within 20 years of developing the disease. This is the highest mortality rate for any psychiatric disease.[18.]

Our attitudes and behaviors toward food can have a profound impact on how our children interact with food. A study of 200 children during their first five years of life showed that those children whose mothers had signs of an unhealthy relationship with their weight had a higher chance of developing eating disorders. Mothers who had dissatisfaction with their bodies, who had excessive dieting or bulimia had an increased chance of having their children develop an altered body image and a resultant eating disorder.[19] In her 2003 book, *Healthy Teens, Body and Soul: A Parent's Complete Guide*, Dr. Andrea Marks describes some adolescent patients as reporting having "pinpoint onset" of their anorexia in response to a hurtful event or comment. Parental opinion, according to Marks and other authors, can have devastating effects on a vulnerable teenager's self-esteem.[20] Repeated negative comments about an at-risk teen's weight or appearance can trigger the cascade of negative self-image and resultant abnormal eating patterns. As parents, it is easy to blame ourselves for our children's illnesses, especially their psychiatric illnesses, but so many of these illness have multiple factors contributing to them. However, as parents, we must be mindful of the influence we hold in our teens' lives and exercise judgment in how our behavior and comments might affect their self-image.

Early recognition and treatment of anorexia nervosa can decrease the death rate from this disease significantly. The aggressiveness of the treatment depends on the progression of the disease and how medically stable the young adult is. In some cases, residential treatment for anorexia is required.

Modalities for treatment include intensive psychological therapy as well as stabilization of the child's weight loss and treatment of any medical conditions such as gastrointestinal disease, liver disease, and cardiac disease which may have developed as a result of prolonged starvation. At times, placement of a feeding tube through the nose into the stomach to provide needed nutrients, as intensive psychological therapy is undertaken, is required. With early recognition and intensive therapy, the death rate from anorexia nervosa can be significantly decreased.

Bulimia nervosa: Bulimia was surprisingly first described in 1979, but is second only to anorexia nervosa as a cause of death in patients suffering from eating disorders. Patients suffering from bulimia are similar to those suffering from binge eating but they engage in purging activities after binge eating to prevent weight gain. These purging activities can involve voluntary vomiting where the young adult will use some mechanism such as sticking her fingers down her throat to induce vomiting. The use of laxatives to induce diarrhea as well as the use of water pills to cause the loss of fluids is also a purging mechanism used by bulimics. A smaller percentage of bulimic patients will engage in excessive exercise in an attempt to feel better about their binge eating. Binge eating as previously discussed may be related to the need to counteract negative feelings about oneself, depression or anxiety. During the binge-eating episode the patient is unable to control their eating and can eat in a frenzied fashion to the point of stomach pain and distress. This is associated with feelings of shame, guilt as well as depression and/or anxiety. The bulimic will then use purging or excessive exercise in an attempt to counteract these negative feelings.

The signs of bulimia include:

- Signs that weight loss, dieting, and control of food are becoming a primary life focus
- Signs of binge eating—the disappearance of large quantities of food from the home, empty wrappers or containers, or food hidden in the young adult's room
- Evidence of purging activity such as disappearance immediately after a meal, signs of vomitus in the bathroom, discarded wrappers or containers, or laxatives or diuretics
- Avoidance of eating around other people

- Appearance of food rituals such as eating only certain types of foods, or abnormal preparation or placement of food on the plate
- Eating limited amounts of food at a meal or skipping meals entirely
- Limiting one's intake of liquids to only water or noncaloric fluids
- Abnormal swelling of the cheeks in the area of the salvia glands due to excessive purging
- Irritation of the hands or knuckles from self-induced vomiting
- Excessive wear to the teeth or staining of the teeth from repeated vomiting
- Extreme mood swings
- Body weight may be normal
- Frequent gastrointestinal complaints such as bloating, increased gas, cramping, and nausea
- Abnormal or missing periods in menstruating girls

Adapted from Warning Signs and Symptoms of Bulimia. National Eating Disorders Association. www.nationaleatingdisorders.org/learn/by-eating-disorder/bulimia/warning-signs-symptoms.
Accessed December 2017.

A high percentage of young adults with bulimia have other psychiatric illnesses. These include mood disorders, anxiety, and substance abuse. Abuse of alcohol, drugs as well as prescription medications is more common in this population that in young adults without eating disorders. Binging and purging of food as well as the overuse of laxatives and diuretics can have devastating effects on every organ system in the body. Repeated forceful vomiting can result in irritation and in some cases significant damage to the feeding pipe (esophagus). Bleeding from tears in the esophagus is one of the causes of death in patients with life-threatening bulimia.

Treatment for bulimia focuses on identifying the other psychiatric illnesses that can contribute to the development of an eating disorder. Without identification and treatment of other underlying psychiatric illnesses that may be present in the bulimic, the success rate for a cure from bulimia is low. The use of antidepressants as well as antianxiety medication coupled with cognitive behavioral therapy has shown some success in the treatment of bulimia. As with anorexia nervosa, inpatient residential therapy may be required to stabilize the condition.

Treatment for eating disorders can be complicated and expensive as medical professionals battle both the psychological and medical effects of eating disorders. As with any chronic illness, involving your primary health care provider as the leader of your child's health care team is essential. All reports from both outpatient and residential providers should be forwarded to them, and they can act as a source of support for you as a parent as you partner with your child on their road to recovery.

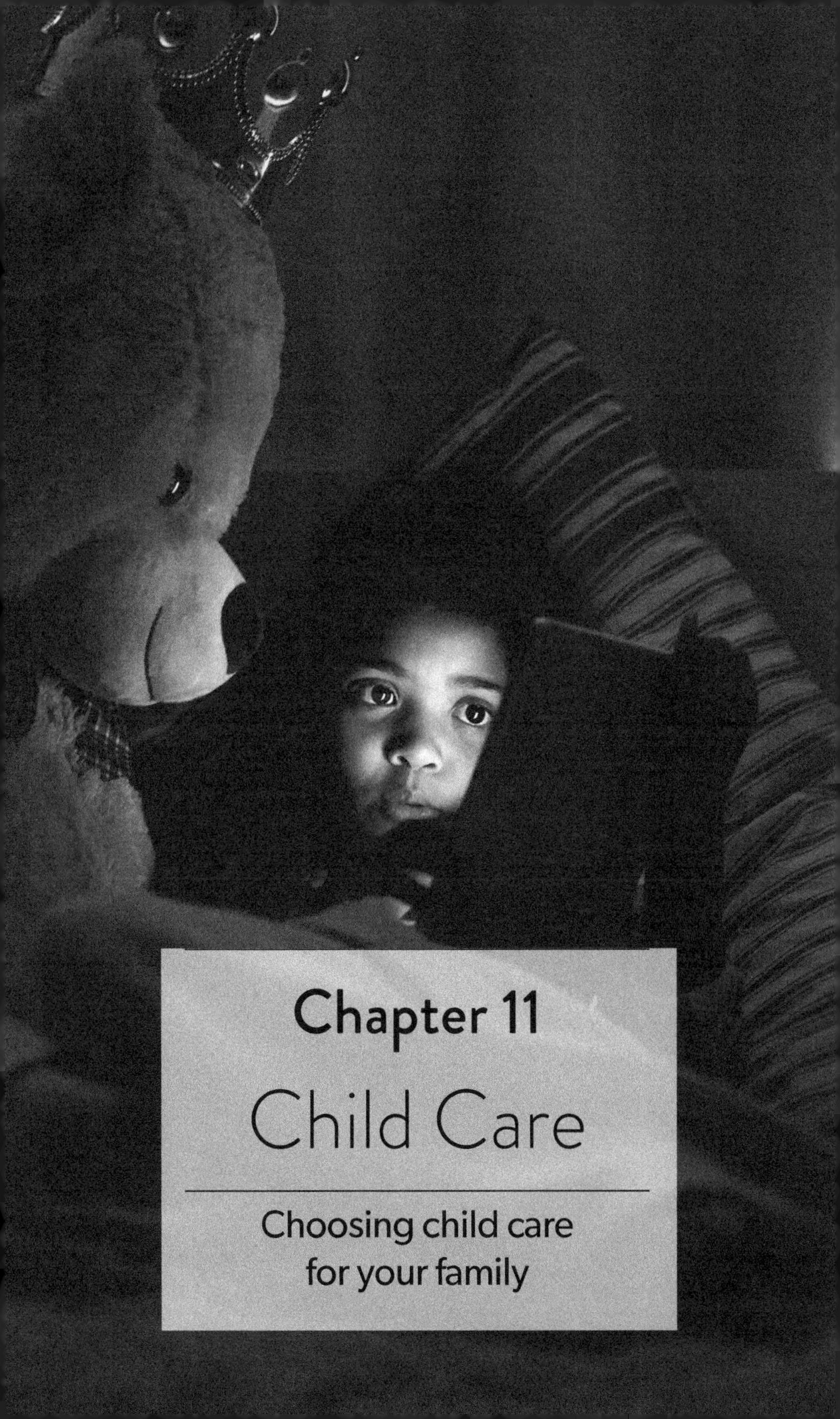

Chapter 11

Child Care

Choosing child care for your family

You and your family must look at your individual situation and assess what type of resources you have

The buzz of the office intercom interrupted my lengthy explanation of how to prepare a two year-old for surgery. The young couple I was addressing sat close together, their wriggling blond-haired boy perched between them.

"Dr. Jones."

The persistent voice of my secretary reverberated through the room from the phone on the wall.

"I think you better pick up, its Vicki."

Vicki had been my babysitter for the past two years. If not for her, I never would have been able to work the hours I did and still have a family.

I picked up immediately.

"Jackie, you know today is the interview at the Presbyterian School. It starts in half an hour. Should I meet you there?"

Terror struck me. How could I have forgotten my son's most important interview of the fall! Having grown up in suburban Long Island in the 1960's, the process of interviewing for nursery school was completely foreign to me. This was not suburban Long Island, however, this was the Upper East Side of Manhattan, where competition for coveted nursery school spots was fierce. I had learned from the other doctors, slightly older than I, how important this process was. The right nursery school meant the right elementary school, the right high school and of course the possibility of Harvard or Yale. My husband thought I had completely lost my mind, but I wasn't willing to take any chances with my first-born son's future. He needed that spot!

"Oh no, Vicki, I completely forgot. Can you get him dressed and I'll meet you there?"

I turned and tried to concentrate on the task of making this family feel comfortable with their decision to proceed with surgery. Luckily, we had been together for almost 20 minutes, so I had already addressed most of their concerns.

"If you have any more questions, please don't hesitate to contact me." I smiled warmly and walked them slowly to the desk. "Please call Mary, my surgical coordinator, whenever you are ready and we will be happy to find a time that works for both of us."

I walked slowly toward my office, rounded the corner and broke into a sprint. Thank God I always dressed up for work and happened to be wearing my favorite suit that day. I grabbed my purse and headed out the back door.

The Presbyterian School was just a few short blocks from my office. I rushed through the crowded New York City streets uttering the frequent refrain, "so sorry, excuse me," as I weaved through the crowd.

I arrived right on time and entered the sun-drenched foyer to find Vicki and my son waiting for me.

"Thank you so much, Vicki, you've saved me again!"

"Of course, Jackie, should I wait or do you want to call me when you're ready?" "Why don't you come back in an hour? I'm sure we will be done by then.

Thanks again."

I grabbed my child's hand and headed toward the reception area. I peeled off his blue coat and was met with a riot of color. An orange shirt and purple-striped pants covering his conservative dress shoes visually assaulted me. My beautiful boy smiled back at me, his tussled curls shinning in the afternoon sun. He looked obviously pleased with his clothing choice.

How could I have forgotten to tell Vicki what to dress him in? I had purchased tweed knickers with suspenders and a beautiful white shirt and socks. It was cute, understated and high fashion in the two to three year-old Upper East Side crowd. I broke into a cold sweat. I looked up to see the round, wrinkled face of the Admissions Director, her gray hair tied in a bun and her roomy skirt and top flowing around her.

"Welcome, young man," said her warm and melodic voice. She moved slowly toward us, and the sweet smell of lavender billowed around her.

"We are so glad you have come to spend some time with us." The gentle, quieting manner of her personality put me and my somewhat shy son immediately at ease.

"It's so nice to meet you, Dr. Jones. We will have a chance to speak later, but for now I would like to speak with this handsome young man."

The Admissions Director held out her hand, and they walked into a brightly lit playroom together. A long half hour passed as I fidgeted on the low green couch that filled the small reception area. I knew in my heart that I was taking this whole nursery school process way too seriously. I couldn't remember even going to nursery school, let alone interviewing for a spot, but there was a part of my brain where doubt thrived. Wasn't it my responsibility to do everything in my power to give my child access to any opportunity available? If that meant having him memorize his address and phone number and wear tweed knickers for his interviews, so be it. Oh no, those tweed knickers! My son sat in his interview at the most prestigious nursery school in New York City with a orange shirt and purple pants. We were doomed.

The door to the playroom opened and my son ran toward me.

"Mom, Mom!" He catapulted across the waiting room, clutching a teddy bear who was wearing a white knit sweater with the words "Presbyterian School" stamped across it's chest.

"Mom, look what I got!" He thrust the teddy bear toward me.

"That's wonderful, sweetie. I'm so happy for you." I smiled and gave him a hug.

"Please join me in my office, and we can have a moment to chat." The warm, wrinkled face of the Admissions Director welcomed us forward.

I settled myself on the roomy couch in her office as my child explored the toys that cluttered the fluffy rag rug of the play space to the side.

"I was so impressed with the time I spent with your son.

He is engaging, smart and rather independent. Kudos to you for letting him express himself. He told me he picked his own clothes today."

I quickly closed my mouth, which had dropped toward my chest at her words.

"Thank you so much. He is a wonderful child," I stammered.

We spent the next ten to fifteen minutes chatting. She slowly rose and turned to engage my son.

"It was so nice to meet you, young man. I hope you enjoyed our visit today?"

My son looked up from the carpet, surrounded by toys, his bear clutched tightly to his chest.

"This was so much fun. Can I come back again?"

Her eyes crinkled and the lines on her weathered face deepened as she smiled back at him.

"We would love to have you visit us again. I hope soon."

She extended her hand and his small fingers intertwined gently with hers.

As we exited the front door, Vicki rounded the corner and waved, a luminous smile brightening her face at the sight of my son. He hurled himself down the sidewalk and into her arms.

"Vicki, look what I got!" He thrust the teddy bear toward her as she covered his shining face with kisses. A pang of jealously always stuck me when I witnessed the closeness of their bond, but I shrugged it off.

She lowered him to the ground and they skipped the last

twenty feet towards me.

"How did it go? I'm sorry about the outfit, but he was pretty insistent about what he wanted to wear today. I figured it wasn't worth upsetting him by getting into an argument."

I gazed at this woman who was such an integral part of my life. Each morning she arrived at 6:30am and enveloped my child in loving arms. The same age as I, we had grown together as I learned so much from her, and, I hope at times, she from me.

Soon after I became pregnant my mother's battle with brain cancer intensified. I alternated weekly trips to her chemotherapy and radiation sessions with visits to my obstetrician for sonograms, blood work and ever increasingly frequent checks on my baby's growth and maturation. I was working 12-hour days, six days per week as I attempted to build a reputation for myself in the competitive New York City medical environment. Exhaustion and stress seemed to be constant companions.

As my 36th week of pregnancy approached, I realized I needed help. I remembered seeing a bulletin board in the waiting area of the post-partum unit just a few floors down from my office. The bulletin board was full of scraps of paper and full-page brochures advertising nanny services. I chose several and began my search. By my 38th week I was becoming desperate. My mother had lapsed into a coma and lay in a hospital bed waiting to die. Finding a nanny became imperative as the reality of caring for this delicate newborn child without the support of my family struck me with terrifying force.

Saturday morning arrived with gusts of cold wind on that early March morning. Vicki and her mother laid their heavy coats on the bench by the front door, slipped off their sneakers and pushed them under the bench.

"No need," I murmured, but they were already settling themselves on the couch, as my husband extended his hand.

My Lamaze instructor had referred Minnie, or "Mama" as everyone called her, to me. Mama was still working for another family but she had brought her daughter Vicki to meet me. We chatted about how Vicki had just moved to the country with two small children but had a large extended family and was more than willing to work the hours I needed. Vicki had a calm personality and a lovely smile. Mama was knowledgeable about childcare, and I figured that by hiring Vicki I had a package deal. How right I was!

We were together along the path of life for over 18 years. Through good times and bad times, through the death of both of our mothers and the untimely loss of her husband. Through the graduation of both of her children from high school and the launch of my boys toward college. It was not always easy, and our styles of parenting did not always mesh, but we worked through our differences together, and I am still so blessed to have her as part of my life.

Child Care

The decision of whether to seek additional care for your child is a personal one. You and your family must look at your individual situation and assess what type of resources you have and if you can "go it alone." There is a select group of couples that are fortunate enough to have one parent stay at home to care for their children. Many parents are forced to choose to either work outside the home or have at-home jobs that do not allow them the time to concentrate on childcare. What options are available?

Staying at Home

How lucky are you to have the financial ability to have one parent stay at home. The advantages of being a stay-at-home parent are obvious. You have unlimited time with your child. You will be the one to see them take their first steps, utter their first words and be there for pick-up and drop-off each day at school. You will get to control how your child is raised and structure how their education advances.

The decision to stay at home should be a joint decision between you and your partner. Are you both committed to having one of you make a drastic change in your lifestyle? This is a discussion that should start during your pregnancy. The vast majority of working parents are afforded maternity and, in some instances, paternity leave. Decide early how you will structure that leave. Will you take time off simultaneously, or will you stager that time off? Will you take time off to prepare for delivery, or will all your time off occur after the baby is born? This is an optimum time to talk together about how you both will care for your child. Do you both feel that staying at home is the right choice for your infant and for your family?

Child care is a 24-7 job, and everyone needs some personal time. How will that be negotiated?

Make a household budget. Make sure you and your partner can afford the loss of one salary and that you both feel comfortable with the changes in your lifestyle that will come from the change in your financial status.

If your financial situation does not allow the complete loss of one salary, can one of you go part-time? Be sensitive to the fact that your partner may not want to take the burden of being solely responsible for supporting the family and perhaps may want to work part-time as well. As with all facets of marriage, negotiation and compromise are vitally important as you enter into this conversation.

Once you have elected to pursue a stay-at-home path, fully utilize the time prior to the delivery of your child. Check out websites for stay-at-home parents and blogs from other parents who have chosen the same path as you. One of the drawbacks of being a stay-at-home parent is the possibility of becoming isolated.

Your child may have become your full-time job but don't forget to interact with other adults and keep your mind engaged and active. Many gyms and community centers provide short-term babysitting for free or for a minimal price. Join a book club in the evening of other parents where the emphasis is on reading short stories, poems or even listening to audio books. Chose any activity that allows you to be an engaged and social adult.

Stay organized. During the first few months of being a stay-at-home parent it may seem like there are not enough hours in the day to care for your newborn, feed you and your partner and make it to the shower once per day. As your baby's schedule regulates you will find more free time for yourself. Plan your day so that both you and your baby are following some schedule. Try to make time once per day to concentrate on yourself. Read the paper for a half hour, lie in a bubble bath, go to the gym. As your baby ages and enters the toddler years think of ways to have them interact with other children. Play dates, library time and gym classes at the local YMCA or community center are all ways to have your child meet other children who are developing at a similar pace as they are. Plan these activities on a master calendar so that you stay organized and engaged.

Choosing to stay at home is no longer limited to just women. A Pew research report in 2016 reported that 17% of the 11 million stay-at-home parents were fathers.[21] The National At-Home Dad Network is a group dedicated to supporting the at-home father. They estimate that almost 7 million fathers are the primary caregivers for their children, meaning they provide reasonably regular care, and that 1.4 million fathers are stay-at-home dads, meaning that they are the daily primary caregiver for their children.[22]

The choice to be a stay-at-home dad is one which must be considered as a family unit. Will this shift in gender roles be difficult on either member of the couple? The Pew report illustrated the gender bias that still exists in our society when men choose what may be considered "non-traditional" roles. The report found that 39% of Americans felt a child was best cared for at-home by their mother, while only 5% felt a child would be better cared for by a stay-at-home father.[23]

Fathers who choose to stay at home will need to find support networks in their community and even nationwide. The National At-Home Dad Network has an informative website and holds an annual convention where stay-at-home dads can network and share the joys and frustrations of the path their family has chosen.

Being a stay-at-home mom has its challenges as well. While stay-at-home mothers are blessed with the joy of being the primary caregiver for their children, they are also plagued by the boredom, loneliness and lack of personal time that many stay-at-home moms report. A 2012 Gallup survey found that a higher percentage of stay-at-home moms report feelings of sadness, anger and worry as compared to mothers who were employed outside the home. This 2012 study found that 28% of at-home mothers reported depression, compared to only 17% of mothers employed outside the home. In addition, lower-income mothers struggled the most with emotional well-being. [24] It is postulated that these feeling of sadness, anger and in some cases depression come from the isolation that can occur when a parent's primary social interaction during the day is with only their children.

Experts believe that the lack of financial independence as well as less personal time contribute to feelings of frustration and isolation.[25]

Stay-at-home parents, both moms and dads, need to recognize the need to care for themselves.

Ways to stay healthy both emotionally and physically include:

1) **Exercise:** The American Heart Association recommends at least 75 minutes per week of vigorous exercise or 150 minutes per week of moderate exercise. They recommend 30 minutes of exercise five days per week to reach these goals. The AHA does not define how or where that exercise should occur, so be creative. Find a gym close by that opens early or closes late or that has childcare. The advantage of a gym is the ability to have social interactions with other adults, even if it is just chatting in the locker room or by the water fountain.

   If your budget is tight, research the YMCA or local community gyms that may be more economical. If joining a gym is impractical for your lifestyle consider a "home gym." This can be as fancy as purchasing a treadmill to as simple as free weights and a jump rope. There are a multitude of apps that provide a routine that fits your fitness level and tracks your progress.

2) **Sunshine and Fresh Air:** Getting outside the house each day is essential to keeping grounded. The daily interaction with other adults as well as the opportunity to get exercise and fresh air is invaluable. This might be as simple as a walk around the block with your child in the carriage to a hike once per week with your infant in a carrier on your back. The important thing is to get dressed, mobilize yourself to be involved in your environment and get outside of your home.

3) **Maximize Your Nutrition:** It is so easy to fall into the

habit of eating whatever your kids are eating. In a perfect world our children would be eating well-rounded, healthy meals three times per day with healthy snacks inbetween and minimal sugar. Let's get real, that probably does not happen in most of our homes. As parents we do the best we can but at times give in to mac and cheese with no vegetables or pizza. The trap is when we get too busy or tired to take care of ourselves. Eating leftovers from your kids plates or resorting to peanut butter and jelly on toast does not lead to a healthy body. More and more grocery stores have salad bars as well as sections of prepared foods.

Big chain supermarkets frequently stock cooked chicken at a reasonable price. Making a large bowl of oatmeal and several hard-boiled eggs at the beginning of the week will make the challenge of a healthy breakfast or lunch when you have no time, easier to deal with. Don't be a martyr, ask your partner to pick up dinner for the two of you once or twice a week on their way home from work. They work hard but so do you, so share the burden.

4) **Find companionship:** Remember you are not in this alone. Many parents have chosen the same path that you have and would love to connect. Make the effort to introduce yourself to other moms and dads at the library, the park and at your children's classes. Be friendly and outgoing and ask them over for coffee and a play date. Having that connection with another

adult is crucial to combatting your feelings of isolation. Develop a group of friends who can be a support network for you. Organize a recurring date to meet and spend time together. Talk about the frustrations you have as well as the joys of being an at-home parent.

If you can't be there...

Many parents are faced with the challenge of caring for their children while pursing employment outside the home. Options for having others care for your child include care by a relative, care by a hired professional or care outside your home. Each have advantages and disadvantages, and the decision on which path you choose should be well-thought out and extensively researched. This needs to, as all major decisions regarding your child should, be a decision that you and your partner make together.

1) **Care by a relative:** Your mother-in-law has offered to watch your newborn when you return to work or your sister is willing to take your two kids during the day when your maternity and/or paternity leave ends. How fortunate for you! There are some issues to consider before you jump into this arrangement though.

   A) The advantages of having a relative care for your child are obvious. You have someone who loves your child and loves you. They are committed, and there will be no awkward phase in trying to get to know them. There will also be no potential for the loss of this valuable person from your child's life. The attachment your child makes to your relative at this stage will be present throughout their life and will hopefully be a grounding and positive outlet for your child as they grow.

You and your relative will share similar cultural values, which will help, as you share the same expectations for what your child will eat, what they will wear and how they will interact with the community you live in. You may be able to save money, as it is unlikely your mom or mother-in-law will ask for an exorbitant wage to care for your child.

B) The disadvantages to having a relative care for your child are also present. Can your relative give you the hours you need to provide adequate care for your child? If you have to try to find additional childcare weekly then that will add a level of stress you don't need. Do you and your relative share a common philosophy for childcare? It will be harder to argue with your mother-in-law about disciplining your children or following a special diet than it will be to tell a hired professional your wishes and assume he/she will follow them. Are you willing to compromise on your views if your relative has strong feelings on how to raise your child? Will your 70 year-old mother have the energy to chase a two year-old around the park for several hours per day and want to have play dates with other 30 year-old moms or caregivers? This might be something she would enjoy but it's best to know your relatives strong points and weak points before you commit.

The issue of whether you should pay your relative for childcare could be difficult. It is unfair to assume that your sister, sister-in-law or cousin is willing to care for your child for free, especially if you are asking for a long-term commitment on their part. You should discuss the subject of paying for their services before they begin caring for your child. You should research current salaries of nannies in your community so you can have a frame of reference to begin your discussion.

While it is unlikely that you and your family member will have a significant difference of opinions in how you should raise your child, there is the possibility that you may not be able to agree on major issues. It will be more difficult to fire a family member and not have it affect your relationship than it would be to fire a professional nanny. It may also strain your relationship if you decide to cut back on the number of hours you require childcare and your family member has come to depend on that income.

Prior to hiring a relative to care for your child ensure that:

1) Your relative can commit to the number of hours you need to make child care as stress free as possible. Will the care occur in your home or their home? If you are late coming home from work, how flexible can they be?

2) Discuss if the other members of their family feel comfortable with the arrangement you are proposing. Will your dad feel his time with your mother is being compromised if she takes on the role of a full-time caregiver for your child? Will this arrangement cause problems in your relationships with other members of your family?

3) Be certain that you and your relative talk about how you will communicate major issues around childcare with each other. Will that be a weekly telephone call or sitting down once every few weeks to discuss the challenges and triumphs you both have as your child grows?

4) The issue of payment should be openly discussed between the two of you. Come to this discussion armed with current salaries and benefits that childcare professionals in your community receive. Be open to revisiting this discussion in 12-18 months as your child ages and becomes more active

and the responsibilities for caring for your child change.

5) Communicate that your relationship with your family member is more important than convenient childcare. Stress with your relative how much you appreciate their involvement in your child's life and remind yourself daily how lucky you are to have relatives who are there for you and your family.

1) **Hiring a Professional to care for your child:**

The vast majority of parents who elect to have their child cared for in their home will hire a professional nanny for that care. The decision to hire at- home help requires you, as a parent, to do your due diligence in researching the qualifications and temperament of the person who will spend more waking hours with your child, in most cases, than you will.

One of the first decisions is whether this professional will live in your home or not. The luxury of having a live-in nanny is tempered by the loss of privacy by having a non-family member in your home. Does your home have a space that your live-in nanny will feel comfortable in? Does your budget allow for the expense of a salary for the live-in nanny as well as the increase in food and resources such as electricity and gas that are part of your household expenses?

Live-in care

A) Au pair services: An au pair is usually a young woman or man who is placed by an employment agency. They most commonly are from a different country, and the amount of time they will commit to spending with you varies. One of the advantages of an au pair is that you, your family and the au pair will learn about each others cultures as you become a part of each others lives. The disadvantages are that you will, in most cases, be unable to meet the person assigned to you in person prior to their arrival.

An au pair is here for a cultural experience and would expect to be considered an "honorary member" of the family, included in family meals and outings. They will generally have less experience than a professional nanny and therefore may require more instruction from you as a parent and employer.

Set clear goals and expectations with your au pair as to what responsibilities you expect them to assume as well as the routine number of hours you expect them to work. Discuss how much advance notice they will need to babysit outside of their routine hours and how much they will be compensated for this extra time. As they are commonly young people discuss acceptable behavior, such as the use of alcohol and cigarettes in your home and if they can have guests, especially overnight guests or guest of the opposite sex, when they are not on duty. Discuss the amount of noise which is tolerable in the house and if you have a curfew for the night before their morning shift. The more that you can discuss issues that may arise early in your relationship, the better experience you both will have.

B) **Professional live-in nanny**: The process of hiring a live-in nanny who may be with you for many years should be a detailed and thorough process. Allow a minimum of six weeks to find the right nanny. Many parents use an employment agency to assist with the search. The advantage of this type of support is that prospective candidates will have undergone a background search and preliminary interview prior to meeting with you. This does not negate your responsibility as a parent to do your own investigation of a potential nanny. There are multiple online services that can add an extra layer of screening to ensure that you have chosen the right candidate. If you choose to find a nanny on your own, ask friends and colleagues for referrals and suggestions. Develop a list of questions and present them to each applicant to see how they would handle different situations. Do your background checks and call all of their references. When you have narrowed your selection to your top two candidates have them return for a second interview.

If you have older children, introduce them to the applicants to see their reaction and how they interact with each other. Show potential applicants the room they will inhabit and discuss if they will be leaving your home on their days off to stay with friends or family.

Once you have chosen a nanny, give them paid time-off to move in and settle into their space. Make sure there is adequate closet and dresser space for their things and that you have no personal items stored in the room that you have reserved for them. Draw up and make sure both of you sign a written contract that should include salary, work hours, responsibilities and whether you will provide insurance. Provisions must be spelled out in the contract for vacations and for an appropriate notice of your nanny terminating their employment with you. In most cases a 60-day notice for both the employer and live-in employee is appropriate.

The decision to hire a live-in nanny is one which should not be taken lightly. Having another caregiver live in your home with you, however, gives you the luxury of an individual who will hopefully become a part of your family and the flexibility of knowing in an emergency someone is always there.

Live-out care:

The more common arrangement for many parents

is to have a nanny care for their child during the day and then have the caregiver return to their own home at night. Having a professional nanny come to your home for childcare, affords you extra time in the morning to spend with your child that would otherwise be spent transporting them to a daycare center. Children who are cared for at home have less exposure to viruses and bacteria than those children in daycare and on average experience fewer episodes of upper respiratory infections during their first year of homecare as compared to children who are cared for in a group setting outside the home.

While a live-out nanny may not be in your home for 24 hours a day, they do spend eight to twelve hours per day alone with your child. The same level of scrutiny of their credentials that you would perform with a live-in nanny should be undertaken. You can use an employment agency or, in the best-case scenario, you can find a candidate through referral from a friend, colleague or neighbor. Interview at least four candidates and narrow your search down to two. You should perform a thorough background search that includes a drug test. Have the candidates return to meet you, your partner and your child. Both you and your partner need to agree that this is the right person for your family. You should then present a written contract with your offer of employment that covers:

1) **Pay Schedule**: Will your nanny's pay be hourly or by the week? What will the pay be for hours worked overtime? Professional childcare employees are covered by the federal Fair Labor and Standards Act and must be paid at least minimum wage and receive overtime pay if they work more than 40 hours per week. Visit the National Domestic Workers Alliance site (www.domesticworkers.org) to learn more about specific laws that apply to domestic workers in your state.

2) **Work hours**: Will your nanny work the same hours five days per week or are there times when you will be home early on a routine basis?

3) **Vacation**: Will you be guaranteeing a certain number of vacation and sick days and will the vacation be paid or unpaid?

4) **Responsibilities**: Cooking, cleaning and childcare should be explicitly described. Will your nanny be cooking only for your child or preparing a meal for the family? Will they need to do food shopping or make a list for you? Will they be doing light cleaning or a heavy clean once every two weeks? Will they be doing your child's laundry or the families'

laundry?

5) **Notice of termination**: Your nanny should give you at least one month's notice if they will be terminating their employment with you. You should give a minimum of two weeks notice if you will no longer need their service, unless there is a cause for termination, in which case it will be immediate.

6) **Taxes**: Taxes can be a source of confusion and anxiety for parents, but it is illegal not to pay taxes for your domestic employee. Provide your nanny with a W-2 form and make sure that you pay the employer share of their taxes. Consider consulting with a tax professional to help ensure that you fulfill your obligation as the employer of a domestic worker.

7) **Insurance**: Your responsibility as an employer concerning insurance should be clearly stated in the contract. Will you be paying for health insurance for your employee or will they be required to obtain health insurance on their own? Some states require that workman's compensation insurance be obtained for a domestic employee. Even if you live in a state where workmen's

> compensation is not required, it is a good idea to consider setting it up. If your nanny is injured at your home, you may be liable to cover their medical expenses. Workman's compensation can help to defray these costs.

A well-thought out contract that covers areas of confusion between you and your nanny will make it less likely that conflict between you and your employee will occur. Discuss with your nanny that you should perform yearly reviews of the contract and performance evaluations. You and your partner should both be present for this evaluation, and you should discuss which areas might need improvement as well as those areas that your nanny has excelled at over the past year. This is also the time to review your expectations of what your nanny's responsibilities will be going forward. Use this discussion as an opportunity for you to adjust what needs to be accomplished in your home. Has your child started school, giving your nanny more free time? Perhaps you can negotiate having your nanny take over some of the cooking or shopping so that you can spend more time in the evening or on the weekend with your family. Don't wait for your yearly conference to discuss issues of concern. Opening lines of communication between the three of you is an important step in forming an alliance that can only benefit your child in the long run.

There may be an adjustment period as you and your nanny get used to each other. If possible, plan to be home for several days after your nanny starts so you have the opportunity to get to know each other and so you can orient them to your home. If you have been using a baby nurse, try to arrange overlap between the two so that both professionals can share information about your newborn. This is a trial period for both you and your nanny, so be open about what you need them to do in order to make you feel comfortable leaving your child with them. This is the time to discuss how in the rare case an emergency occurs, it should be dealt with. You should place a list of important contacts as well as the number for your local poison control center in a visible location. You, your partner's and the pediatrician's phone numbers should all be entered into your nanny's phone. Discuss who should be contacted if you and your partner are unavailable. Is that person a trusted friend or relative? That number should be entered into your nanny's phone as well.

Medical Preparedness

Both you and your nanny want to have the skills needed to deal with any emergencies. There are several companies that provide online and in-person childcare training. One of the most recognized national organizations is the American Red Cross. They provide classes in infant care and childcare as well as classes in First Aid and Cardiopulmonary Resuscitation (CPR) of infants and children.

Their childcare course teaches basic childcare skills such as holding and feeding an infant, child behavior and discipline and home safety. They also have classes in water safety, which you should have your nanny attend if you expect them to supervise your child at the pool or beach.

Download the American Red Cross' guides to "Baby Sitting Basics," "A Baby Sitters Handbook" as well as their "Emergency Reference Guide." Their "Emergency Reference Guide" has a pre-printed sheet to list all your important contact numbers as well as instructions on dialing 911 and how to contact the national poison control emergency hot line. It has a quick reference guide on how to deal with common emergencies such as insect bites, cuts, bruises and even what to do if your child's tooth is knocked out. Their guides can be accessed and downloaded at www.redcross.org/take-a-class/babysitting-child-care.

A class in infant or child CPR is a necessity for any professional childcare worker. This class must be taken in person, and refresher courses should be taken every three years. Keep your nanny's certificate on file and remind them when they need a refresher course. Consider having all the adults in your family register for a CPR class. The skills you learn could help to save your child's life.

You and your nanny should go through your medicine cabinet and review what medication can be given and for what symptoms. If you would like to be called prior to the administration of any medication, make that clear. Do not store unused medications in your medicine cabinet and be sure to store narcotics or more dangerous substances, such as cardiac medications and blood thinners, in a secure location, such as a locked medicine chest. If your child requires daily medication, or medication for an acute illness has been prescribed, review the correct dose and how to administer it. If the medication is in liquid form, consider getting extra syringes from the pharmacy and preloading them. Put out the daily dose and carefully mark it. Do not leave medications, including over the counter medications, in a location that your child can access. Use only medication bottles with child-safe caps.

Put a medication check-off list in a prominent place and have your nanny and any other adult who administers treatment mark off the date and time the medication was given. Prior to surgery many children must refrain from the use of non-steroidal medications, such as Advil, Motrin, aspirin and vitamins. Remove these substances from your medicine cabinet and discuss with all adults who care for your child what restrictions on medications are in place. After surgery, review with your nanny and family members when they can again give over the counter medications as well as the use of any prescription medications.

Safety-proof your home. This process should start before your child becomes mobile and should be a joint effort between you and your child's caregiver.

Steps to Take:

1) Install gates to dangerous areas, such as the kitchen and stairs.
2) Cover all outlets and hang curtain cords at a height that your child can not access.
3) Keep cords to lights, televisions and computers tightly

wrapped and stowed behind furniture. Every year there are deaths recorded of children crushed by objects in their home that they have pulled onto themselves.

4) Install corner guards and bumpers on the sharp corners of coffee tables. Have both you and your nanny enforce the rule of no climbing on furniture that may tip over or be high enough for a fall to cause injuries.

5) Install cabinet latches on all kitchen drawers and cabinets and do not allow your toddler or crawling infant unsupervised access to your kitchen when you are cooking.

6) Turn down the water temperature to less than 120 degrees to avoid the risk of scalding.

7) Never leave any child alone in the bath for even a few minutes. Accidents can happen in seconds.

8) Keep guns securely locked away.

9) Keep sharp tools and chemicals, such as cleaning products, in cabinets with child proof locks.

Your caregiver should be your ally in working to make your home a safe and enjoyable place for the whole family.

Delegating Medical Responsibility to your Nanny

Our nannies become the surrogate parents to our children, so there may be times when they are required to deal with medical situations in our absence. This can range from routine doctor visits to dealing with trips to the hospital for unexpected emergencies. The best preparation to ensure that these visits go well is communication between you, your nanny and your child's primary healthcare provider.

Prior to returning to work, discuss with your pediatricians' office what their policy is on a non-family member accompanying your child to the office. In my office we must have on file a written, signed consent from a parent allowing a specific person to accompany their child to a visit.

What should be included in a Parental Consent form:

1) A statement that allows your nanny to make medical decisions for your child. A statement such as "I grant permission for my child's caregiver (list your caregivers full legal name) to make medical decisions and authorize treatments for my child" should suffice.

2) List your child's full name, date of birth and any pertinent medical history, such as allergies to medications and any prior surgery.

3) List your contact information, including your full name, address andphone number.

4) Sign and date the form and have a witness sign the form.

A copy of the form should be kept on file at your pedia-

These questions should include:

1) **State License:** Be sure to examine their state certificate and ask how often a state regulator visits the center.

2) **Medical Preparedness:**
   - A) Are staff members trained in infant and child CPR?
   - B) Does the center administer routine medications such as Acetaminophen or Non-Steroidal Medications, such as Advil or Motrin? What is the policy for administering these medications?
   - C) If your child is required to take prescription medication during the day will the center administer that medication?
   - D) Does the center have an affiliation with a local hospital? If your child is injured at the center will a staff member stay with your child at the hospital until you arrive?

3) **Background Checks**: Have all administrators and staff at the center undergone background checks and drug testing?

4) **Staff:**

   - A) Ask about credentialing and the educational background of the staff. Do any of the staff members have degrees in early childhood education?

B) What is the ratio of staff members to children and what is their turnover rate?

C) What percentage of the staff speaks English, or your native language, as their primary language?

5) **Cleanliness**: What is the cleaning schedule? It is recommended that the center's bathrooms, floors and tables be cleaned daily and that carpets be cleaned monthly. Toys, both soft and hard, should be cleaned daily, and climbing equipment and larger structures, such as dollhouses, should be cleaned weekly.

6) **Sickness**: What are the center's rules about when your child must stay home for an illness? Many centers require a child to stay out of the center until they have been fever-free for 24 hours.

7) **Educational Curriculum**: What educational programs does the center have in place? Are there any formal assessments of your child's language development and educational progress? Are there opportunities to meet with your child's primary provider to get updates on their development

as well as their educational strengths and weaknesses?

8) **Philosophy**: Does the center's philosophy match your own? Is religion a part of the program? If you are raising your child as a vegetarian, can their diet be accommodated?

9) **References:**Is it possible for you to contact other parents whose children are attending the center to get references? Call the Better Business Bureau and consult online sights such as Yelp, Google and local parent blogs to check the reputation of the center.

Once your have narrowed your choice down to two centers, revisit each center during the day to see how caregivers interact with the children. Once you feel comfortable with the center obtain a contract and take your time to review it thoroughly. It should clearly state the cost of care, the hours of operation of the center and the maximum number of children in your child's age group. There should be a clause allowing you to cancel the contract without cause with a maximum 30-day notice period. Inquire if there are any behaviors on your child's part that would cause the center to terminate your contract. The grounds for termination of your child should be clearly spelled out and include a warning as well as an approximate time period for you to address the concerning behavior.

Family-Centered Childcare:

Family-centered childcare can be an attractive option for some families. There are usually fewer children in a family-centered program, and the environment may be more cozy and intimate. They are also commonly less expensive than commercial childcare centers. Family-centered organizations will usually take care of children of differing ages, so your child will have the opportunity to interact with children in varying developmental stages. This scenario is more like the interactions they would experience at home.

The concern with family-centered programs is that they are not required to go through the same rigorous licensing process as a commercial childcare center. Each state has different requirements for family-operated centers. Some states license these centers, whereas others only require certification. Check your state's requirements by visiting the website of the National Resource Center for Health and Safety in Child Care and Early Education.

Tour the facility and look for signs that the home is well maintained, clean and safe. Are all outlets covered? Do cords or wires dangle too low? Do they have appropriate safety gates? Are the walls freshly painted so that your child has no opportunity to ingest chipped paint? Open the refrigerator. Is it clean and stocked with appropriate snacks for children? Look under the sink. Do you see any signs of rodent droppings or insects?

Questions you should ask on your tour:

1) **Licensure**: Is the center licensed and

how frequently does the state visit, if it is licensed? Is the center a member of the National Association for Family Child Care (NAFCC)? The NAFCC is a non-profit organization that accredits family childcare centers.

2) **Medical Preparedness:**

A) Does the center have a first aid kit? Do they administer medications, either over the counter or prescription?

B) Is the staff member trained in infant and child CPR? How often do they update their certification? A minimum of every three years is recommended.

C) If a child needs to be transported to the emergency room, who will go with the child and who will stay with the other children?

3) **Other Adults in the home**: Who will have access to the children during the day? Do other adults live in the home or visit routinely? Have all persons who come in contact with your child on a regular basis undergone a background check?

4) **Sickness**: What are the policies for when your child is sick? When must they refrain

from attending childcare?

5) **Backup**: If the primary caregiver in the center becomes sick, what backup is available? Does the center close for vacations or any holidays? If there was a sudden emergency requiring the caregiver to leave the facility, what type of backup would be in place?

6) **Cleanliness**: How often are the toys and bathrooms cleaned? How often is the rug cleaned?

7) **References**: Can you speak to the other families whose children attend the center? Research the center on the web and parenting blogs. You can also call the Better Business Bureau to ensure that there have been no complaints registered about the center.

Once you feel comfortable with a family-based center, visit it unannounced. Do the children look well-cared for and clean? Are there age appropriate toys or are the toddlers planted in front of the television? If you feel comfortable with what you see and would like to move forward, ask for a contract. Be sure it lists the costs, hours of operation and refund policy if the center was to close for an unexpected illness or emergency. If the center does not supply contracts, write up a letter addressed to the primary caregiver, listing the issues you feel are vital and ask the center's primary caregiver to sign, date and return it to you. Make a copy for them and keep a copy in your files. Ensure that the letter or contract clearly states the provisions for cancellation on either of your parts. You should have a 30-day notice period to cancel without cause; the center should give you a minimum 60-day cancellation period without cause. Ask the center if there is any behavior on your child's part that would trigger cancellation of the contract. Cancellation for cause on your part should occur immediately.

The choice of a commercial childcare center versus a family-centered childcare center is a personal one. Each option will have advantages and disadvantages, and your choice should be based on your economic situation, how convenient each center is to your work and home and how comfortable you feel with the setting of each center. The most important factor is the safety of your child, followed by a warm, nurturing and supportive atmosphere. Take into account how your child will grow in the environment and whether you feel comfortable switching to a larger more educationally stimulating environment as your child ages. Start the process as early as possible, even before you deliver, so that there is one less stressor in your life as you and your partner navigate your new role as parents.

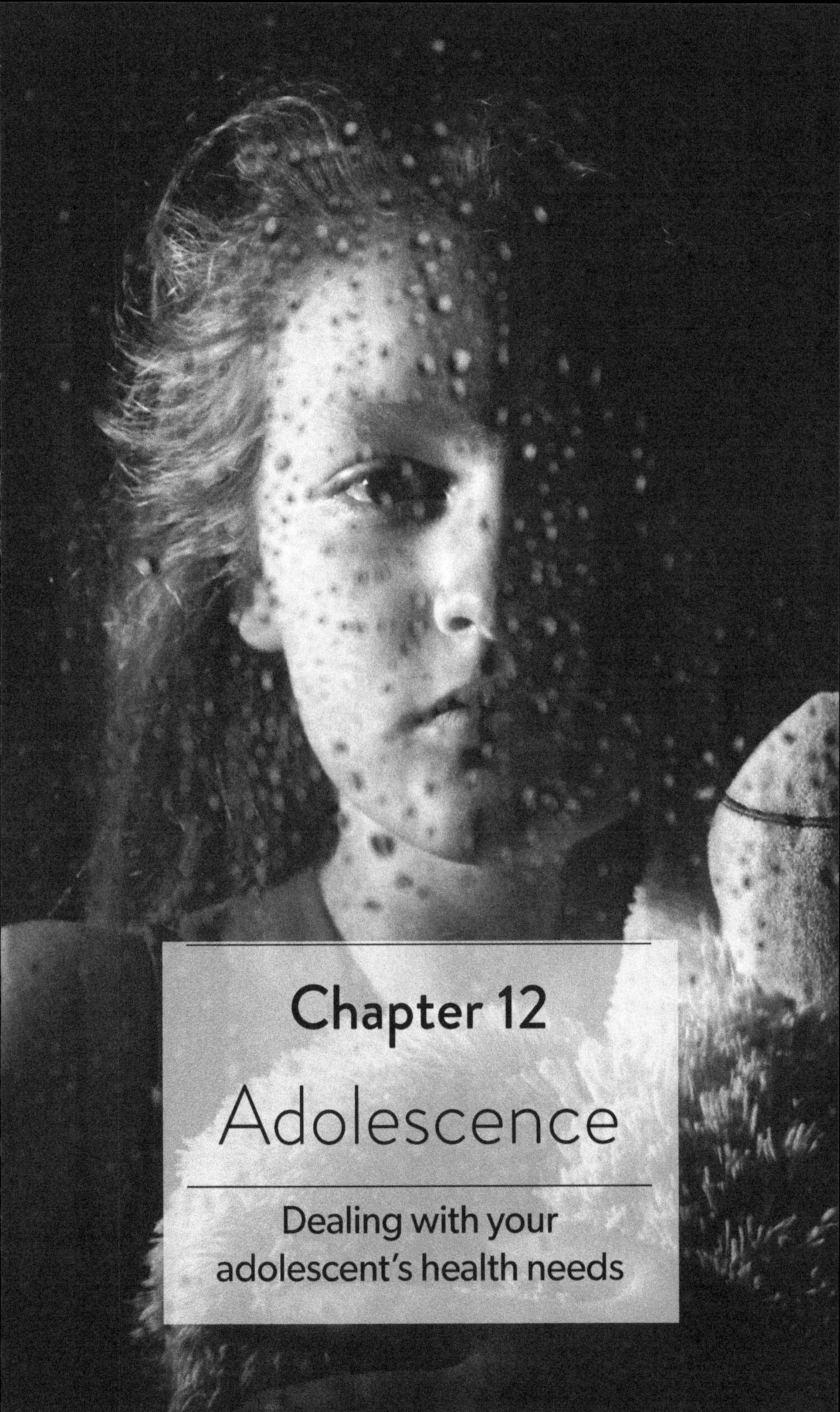

Chapter 12

Adolescence

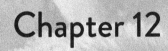

Dealing with your adolescent's health needs

As your child ages, it is important to respect their need to be involved in decisions regarding their care.

I sat perched on the small stool in my exam room looking at Mary—a junior at a New York City high school—slumped over in my examination chair. This was the third time this week she had been at a doctor's office with complaints of a sore throat and ear pain. Her pediatrician, who I knew well and respected as an excellent physician, had been exhaustive in his search for a cause. He had called me earlier that day feeling somewhat frustrated that he could not pinpoint the cause of her discomfort. He told me she had missed two weeks of school and was concerned that stress was a major contributing factor. But, he wanted my input on the best course of treatment.

Mary's mother sat next to her on a small stool—legs crossed, arms tightly folded in her lap, her mouth a thin, hard line across her chiseled face. She emitted anxiety.

"Mary, tell me a little bit more about what's been going on," I asked, my attention focused on the young woman in front of me.

As I do with all teenagers, I gave her the opportunity to take responsibility for her care, instead of her parent.

Her mother answered immediately.

"It's her throat. She has been in such pain for the past week," she said. "We need to fix this immediately. She needs to get back to school."

I turned towards her mom to acknowledge her comments and, most importantly, her fears and frustrations.

"Absolutely. I understand this is a critical time for Mary, and we will work together to get her feeling better as soon as possible."

I turned again toward Mary.

"Mary, tell me what's been going on."

"I'm really not sure why my throat is hurting," she said. "I've tried everything—lozenges, honey, lemon—and it just hurts so badly. Every time I swallow it feels like there is a huge ball in my throat."

"Tell me a little bit about how long this has been going on for," I probed.

"It's been going on for two weeks. Finals start next week and I just can't afford to miss any more school," she said.

We talked more about her history and how frustrated she felt. Her mother tried interjecting every few minutes, but I continued to keep the focus on Mary. As the minutes passed, I could feel Mary relaxing a bit and opening up about her concerns.

"Mary and mom, this is so helpful," I said. "Let's take a look at your throat and try to find a way to make you feel better."

Mary's mom tensed in her seat. I reassured her that I would explain each step of the exam.

I lowered my voice to a quiet whisper so Mary would concentrate on my voice, not my actions. Her mother covered her eyes and leaned over with her head in her lap. Mary and I continued to concentrate on each other and she was easily able to tolerate the small scope I gently passed through her nasal cavity to examine the upper and lower portions of her throat.

It was red and inflamed. There lay the cause of her pain in the back of her throat, where the swallowing passage began. Following the exam, Mary let out a sigh. I leaned over to assure her mom she had done well.

"I think I have found the cause of your throat pain," I said to Mary with a smile, hoping that my calm demeanor would help her and her mother both to relax.

"The back of your throat is irritated and it appears to be from acid washing over your voice box. The acid comes from your stomach and is mostly secondary to changes in your diet and stress."

"Are you sure doctor? Can't this just be fixed with a course of antibiotics?" Mary's mother asked, looking shocked at my diagnosis.

I spent the next several minutes discussing gastroesophageal reflux or heartburn that can produce symptoms of severe sore throat, if left untreated. We discussed how stress could be playing a large role in Mary's symptoms and how Mary and her mother could help to address that stress. We discussed modifications to Mary's diet and the use of medications for a few weeks, to help decrease acid production and throat pain as she worked on her diet and her stress.

Mary promised to call me in the next several days to tell me how she was feeling. We set up an appointment to see each other in three weeks. As Mary and her mom proceeded to the desk, I called her pediatrician to discuss the diagnosis, and how he would follow up with Mary and her mother over the next several days to ensure they understood our conversation, and felt they could comply with my recommendations.

Teenagers are a species unto themselves. The rage of hormones, the lack of confidence in their rapidly-changing bodies, and their need to develop independence from their parents can often make teenagers difficult to understand and at times difficult to deal with. Understanding their need for independence and their need to have a larger role in caring for their own bodies will make your interactions with them less stressful for you both.

Choosing a health-care provider for your teen: As your child ages, it is important to respect their need to be involved in decisions regarding their care. During their 14th or 15th year physical, observe the way they interact with their health-care provider. Do they seem comfortable engaging with their physician? Does the pediatrician/primary care provider give them the opportunity to answer their question while you are not in the room?

Is there a discussion about age-appropriate vaccinations and the implications of declining or accepting these vaccinations?

If you notice your child is uncomfortable following the visit, it is okay to ask them about how they feel. You can ask if they feel comfortable discussing their concerns with the pediatrician and if they think this is the right fit for them. Also ask if the physician answered all of the questions they had. It is likely that you will not receive any information from this initial conversation, but you will be opening avenues for the discussion.

If your teenager brings up the issue again, be open to their thoughts. Your pediatrician may have been an excellent fit for you, but not what your child needs as they transition into adulthood.

Options for adolescent care

Pediatric care: Continuing with your child's pediatrician is the common choice for most teenagers. The vast majority of pediatricians are well versed in transitioning to the care of a teenager that requires a new relationship with their physician. A relationship where trust and confidentiality are important hallmarks. Your adolescent must feel safe in their new relationship with their pediatrician and see them as an advocate for their needs. To foster this relationship your pediatrician's focus must be on your teen during their visits. Don't feel hurt or abandoned, your pediatrician is there for you as a parent as well but building a trusting relationship with your child can only help both you and your child in the long run.

Adolescent care: Pediatricians specializing in adolescent care are another option as your child ages. The American Academy of Pediatrics defines adolescent pediatricians as health-care providers who care for children ages 11 to 24. These physicians may be general pediatricians who have elected to specialize in adolescent health, or health-care providers who have obtained additional training in the care of adolescent patients.

Fellowships in adolescent medicine are commonly three years long, after a physician completes their basic pediatric training.

These health-care providers are specially trained to address the emotional and physical challenges unique to adolescence.

If your child is struggling with more complex problems such as mental health issues, an eating disorder, addiction, or academic or social issues, an adolescent physician can help you address these issues as a family.

The Society of Adolescent Health and Medicine (SAHM) has a website to help locate adolescent health-care providers. SAHM also has an app for smartphones that allows families to access resources to help address and manage issues that are relevant to the needs of adolescents and their families.

Primary care physician: A primary care physician cares for children as well as adults, thus can care for your entire family. They offer the advantage of a continuum of care and the ability of your child to continue their care into adulthood. Be sensitive to the fact that your teen may not want to share a physician with you. This is an opportunity to open a dialogue with your teen about their thoughts and needs for a health-care provider moving forward. Respect their wishes if they seem appropriate, and be respectful in your discussions with your child if their request seems unreasonable—and provide other suggestions instead.

The American Academy of Family Physicians and local hospitals are good resources for locating a family physician who is right for your child and your family.

Doctor's visits with your teenage child: As your child transitions into their teenage years, they face the challenge of moving toward independence. Ask them when their schedule might allow them to see their doctor for a checkup. Giving them ownership in the process may help foster cooperation and involvement in their care. Once an appointment has been made, have your teen put it on their calendar. A day or two before the appointment, ask them how they plan on getting to the appointment. If you accompany them to the office, encourage your teen to interact with the staff and introduce themselves.

This is an important step in letting them take ownership of their visits.

Ask your teen if they want you to accompany them into the exam room, and if they feel comfortable discussing any concerns they may have about their health with you in the room. If you do accompany them into the exam room, give them the chance to interact with their physician prior to your volunteering any information. If they are feeling shy or would prefer not to participate in the discussion, it is appropriate to voice your understanding of the problem and concerns. As with all stages of your child's life, not projecting your anxiety and fears into the discussion will help your teen deal more effectively with their own anxieties surrounding their health.

Once the physician has obtained a history, ask your child if they would like you to leave the room for the examination.

Be sure to respect their wishes, and ask if you can return after the examination is complete. If you get the response "I don't care," from your teen, it could be a sign that your presence is appreciated. If your child is a minor, you have every legal right to be in the room during the visit, but respecting your child's wishes will buy you something priceless: an open and trusting relationship.

If the physician gives treatment recommendations, repeat the instructions out loud with your child and the physician. This ensures that there are no misunderstandings regarding how medication should be administered and if there should be any changes in your child's lifestyle. If you feel that the diagnosis might affect their activity, be open and discuss this with your child and their physician.

In the event of an illness or accident, review when your child can return to school and what extracurricular activities they can engage in. Discuss with the physician if your child should refrain from going out after school or in the evening, or if they should refrain from exposure to "screens" such as phones, computers, and television. Discuss how long these restrictions should remain in place. Give your child the opportunity to ask as many questions as they need to before you leave the office. It is vitally important for them to understand the rationale behind the recommendations for a lifestyle change, and the ramifications of not following them.

If medication is prescribed, review when and how it should be taken with the physician in the room. Can it be taken on an empty stomach, or is food required? If the timing of the medication seems impractical to you, such as four times a day for a busy junior in high school, speak up and discuss with the physician alternatives that would work with your child's schedule. If there are no alternatives to a medication that requires administration during school hours, have the pediatrician explain to your child how to take the medication during the day.

In a busy pediatrician's office, if the physician does not have the time to review these strategies in depth, ask if a nurse can spend time discussing options instead. Remember, suggestions to teenagers are sometimes better received when they come from someone other than their parent.

If additional testing is required—such as blood test and X-rays—be sure to allow your teenager the chance to discuss what information will be obtained by these tests. If they are again uninterested in asking these questions, respect their independence but make sure they understand the importance of having these tests completed. If you feel you don't understand the importance of further testing, be sure to ask questions to help you adequately explain the issues to your child, if they decide to ask you about it on the way home. Don't push their involvement; rather, become an ally and resource to them.

Realistic expectations for dialogue with your teenage child: Even the most open and connected teenager may have issues in their life that they want to keep private. Dealing with concerns over sexuality, body image, and where they socially fit in can be challenging for teens. Allowing your child a safe space to discuss these issues is crucial. If your physician has the opportunity to develop a personal relationship with your child, their office can serve as a safe space. Allowing that relationship to develop means removing yourself as a barrier to create an honest and open discussion. Assuming that your child will never touch alcohol, cigarettes, or engage in any type of sexual behavior in their teenage years age is unrealistic.

While these behaviors may cause you to feel helpless, upset, or frustrated, your pediatrician can have an open discussion around the consequences of risky behavior and how to deal with peer pressure around activities their friends may be pursuing. Allowing the space for these discussions to occur requires trusting that your child will listen to advice from their physician, and that your pediatrician will be able to establish a relationship for healthy, open dialogue. This does not lessen your responsibility as a parent to discuss these issues with your child—it just gives your child another avenue of support to help manage the stresses of adolescence and adulthood.

College preparedness: College is the first time many teenagers will take responsibility for their actions without the safety net of their parent's daily oversight. From getting up for classes, doing their laundry, and managing their time, the stresses of college are manyfold. As you help navigate the health-care responsibilities of college with your child, there are several issues that must be addressed.

Discuss with your child and your pediatrician if additional

vaccinations are recommended. These can include a tetanus booster, the meningitis vaccination, as well as a vaccine for human papillomavirus—a virus that can be sexually transmitted and can increase the risk of cervical cancer and venereal warts. If your child takes medication on a daily basis ask for a three month supply and fill the prescription just before leaving for college.

Most colleges require an up-to-date physical prior to enrollment. Try to schedule this in the spring of your child's senior year of high school, before the camp rush at pediatrician's offices and before your child's schedule become too hectic. Keep a copy of the physical exam for your files.

Ensure that your pediatrician explains to your child how student health services operate on campus. Discuss that in the event of an emergency, the campus health clinic or 9-1-1 should be utilized. If your child is sick, reaching out to their pediatrician or visiting student health services is advisable. Let your student know that if they feel the care they are receiving from an on-campus health-care provider is inadequate, or if they are not feeling better, they can call their pediatrician's office to discuss their concerns.

An open dialogue should occur at this visit with your child and their health-care provider about the importance of granting a release of medical information from the college to their primary care provider and any specialist, who may need to interact with the health services at their school. A release of medical information form should be filled out and signed for each health-care provider who should be granted access. These forms can be mailed to health services when the annual physical form is submitted. A copy should be retained for your files.

Once your child is settled in on campus, help them find the closest pharmacy to their dorm or apartment. Take the time to register your child at the pharmacy and leave their insurance information along with a credit card on file. Both you and your child should store this information in your phones in the event that medication is prescribed while your child is away at school. If you live in a state where electronic prescriptions are required, supply your pediatrician's office with this number so that renewal of prescriptions can also be accomplished in a timely fashion.

If your child has a serious health condition that requires frequent monitoring, you may want to consider developing a relationship with a primary care provider or specialist close to your child's school, as on-campus health services may not be equipped to deal with more complicated medical problems. You and your child can arrange this visit early in the school year. Your pediatrician at home, the college health services center, or a local hospital may be able to supply you with names of competent physicians near the college.

Communication is the hallmark to a healthy parent-teenager relationship. Respecting their need for independence while also setting appropriate boundaries that you feel are necessary for their continued growth and development are essential to being a responsible parent.

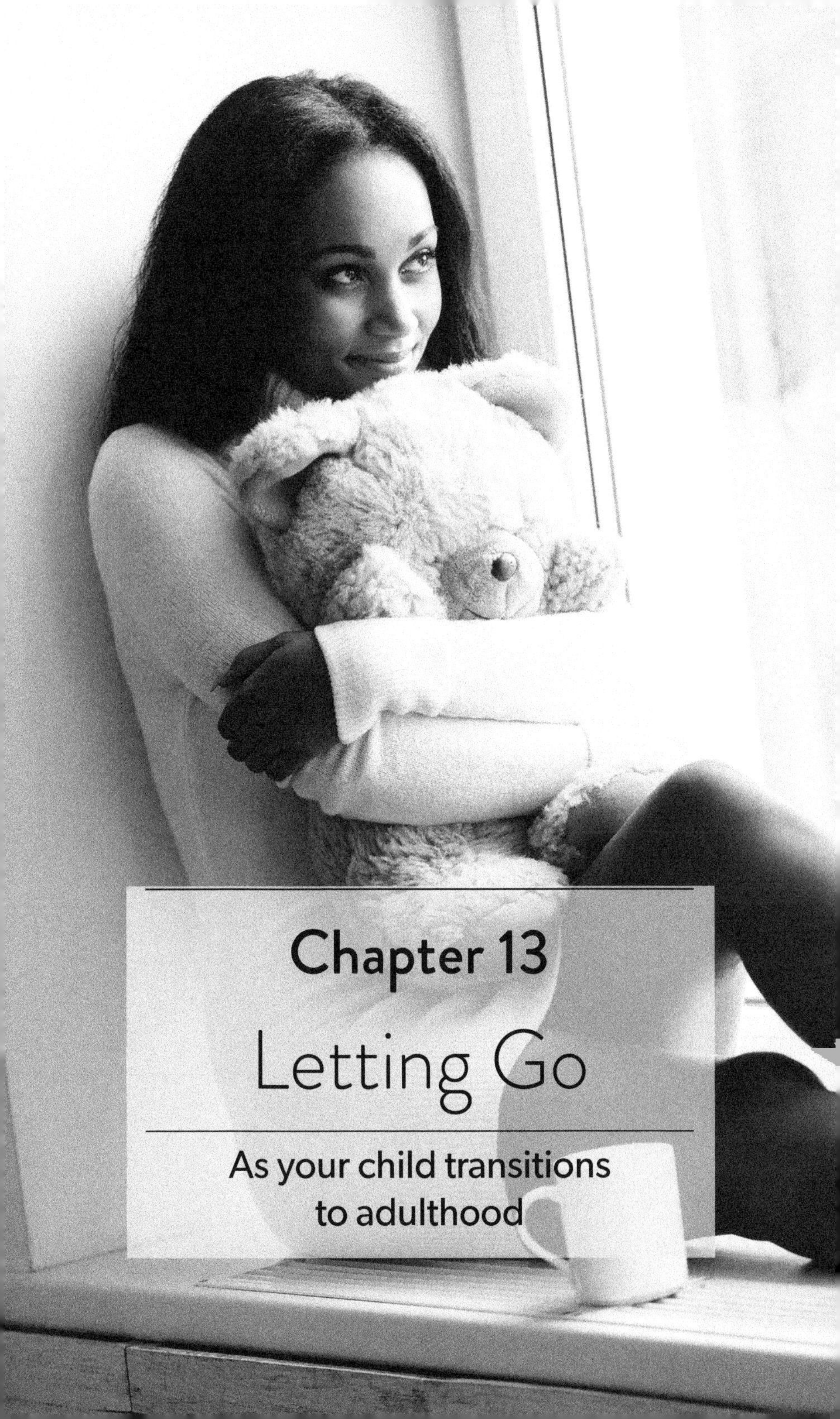

Chapter 13
Letting Go

As your child transitions to adulthood

There is no magic switch that parents can flick on, allowing us to accept that the child we have nurtured, protected, and guided is now a self-sufficient adult.

The shrill ring of the bedside phone pierced the depths of my sleep. Although I was accustomed to waking up abruptly in the middle of the night as a pediatric surgeon, I made sure to grab it before it woke my husband, sleeping next me.

"Hello. Dr. Jones. Can I help you?" I asked, as my brain switched to doctor mode and I struggled to clear the cobwebs of sleep.

"Dr. Jones, I am sorry to call you. This is Dean Reynolds from your son's college."

I stopped breathing and shot upright in bed.

"I'm sorry to call but there has been an accident and your son is in the city hospital. He is stable but I think you should come now."

"Of course, I'm on my way," I said without hesitation.

I jumped out of bed and dressed myself quickly in the neon glow that emanated from my alarm clock. I felt numb and cold as the icy tendrils of fear crept from my stomach to my brain.

"John, John," I shook my husband until his eyes fluttered open. "I have got to go. There's been an accident at school. You stay here. I'll call the babysitter to come. Take the first train in the morning and meet me. I'll call you as soon as I know something. "

Control and action were how I have always dealt with crisis in my life, and this February night was no different. The usual two-hour trip to my son's college was accomplished in 60 minutes. The memory of that drive is a blur, but if there's one thing I do remember, it is being thankful that the police did not follow me. Stopping was not an option.

I arrived at the city hospital and parked out front. I strode into the emergency room and arrived at the triage desk.

"Good evening, I'm Dr. Jones. I need to see my son—now," I said, looking at the nurse with steely determination. Neither she nor the walls that separated me from my child would stand in my way. She glanced at the computer screen and back at me.

"I'm sorry, the doctors are with him now," she said. "Please take a seat we will call you when they are ready to talk to you."

"I'm sure you must be mistaken," I said. "I'm his mother and I need to see him now."

Again, she told me to take a seat.

I felt beads of sweat beginning to form on my forehead. I was afraid I might start screaming any second.

"Get me the nursing supervisor now," I said.

The security guard approached me.

"Is there a problem?" he boomed.

"It's okay, Jake," the triage nurse said. "She's going to sit down and we will call her when the doctors are ready."

I lowered myself into the nearest chair, perched on the edge as I began my vigil. An hour passed and I approached the nurse's station again. She looked up from her computer.

"I'm waiting to see my son," I said. "Can you please see how long it might be?"

I got the same response. She told me to have a seat, and that the doctors would call as soon as they could. She smiled a kind smile and returned to her computer. Fear, rage, and frustration overwhelmed me.

But again, I sat down, and tried to remain calm. Deep breathing and trying to relax were the only things that kept me from tackling the security guard and forcing my way into the emergency room. I closed my eyes and tried to concentrate on slow, even breaths.

I awoke stiff and cramped as the sun poured in through the grimy windows of the city hospital. I rose from my seat, and yet again, approached the nurse's station. A new, younger nurse looked up at me as I leaned heavily on the desk.

"I'm Dr. Jones. I have been waiting to see my son. Can you please see if I can go in?"

"Oh, yes. The doctor came out about two hours ago but you were sleeping and we didn't want to wake you."

I understand now how crimes of passion occur. It was all I could do to keep myself from reaching across the desk and shaking some sense into this obviously flawed human being.

I controlled myself.

"Well, I'm ready to go in. May I see my son now?"

Finally, I did.

The next 18 months were a journey of recovery for us both. I learned to trust that those caring for my son would help him find his path, and I learned the art of taking each small victory as a big step along the path to recovery.

There is no magic switch that parents can flick on, allowing us to accept that the child we have nurtured, protected, and guided is now a self-sufficient adult. The process of letting go takes time and work. But eventually, you will, and accepting that mistakes are inevitable will help you to navigate your new role in your young adult's life.

Your rights as the parent of a legal adult: Most medical offices will let you make an appointment for your adult child. I usually suggest consulting with your child prior to making an appointment. Most young adults have busy lives and you will need to coordinate their schedules with any appointments you will have made. If they "buy-in" by making the effort to find a specific time for the appointment or scheduling the appointment themselves, it is more likely they will be on time and involved in the appointment.

Speak to your young adult about joining them for their appointment. Do not automatically assume that you will have access to their physician. As you navigate your new role in their life, be sensitive to the fact that they are forging their own path towards independence and may want the opportunity to interact with their physician on their own. If you are permitted by your child to join them in the exam room, please remember that you are an invited guest and should respect your child's independence as they interact with their physician. Allow them to discuss their history and their concerns. There may be some sensitive issues that the physician will need to discuss. Leave the room without an argument or attitude, if you are asked by either your child, the physician or support staff to do so.

If your child will need to undress to be examined, allow them the privacy to do so. During the visit, you may have questions you would like answered or clarified by the physician. Ask your child if it is permissible to ask questions. If they say no, respect their decision. If your child is away at school, consider asking them and their physician if you can be listed as an alternative contact. You can assure your child that they will be the primary contact if they so desire, but that you will be available as a backup. A written consent form is required to allow their physician to speak to you. (Fig. 4). Ask your child to complete it at this visit.

Out of respect, only contact your child's physician with their permission. You should act as a secondary form of communication with any of your child's health-care providers. Be mindful that some young adults do not want to take on the responsibility of their own care and will gladly relinquish that chore to you. Be supportive and slowly transition the process of taking over these tasks to them over time. Be communicative and assure they are part of the process and as involved in their care to the greatest extent they are able. Your role is to be there for them, but also to foster independence.

Your rights as the parent of a college-bound student: The day has finally come when your pride and joy will leave home and transition to independence at college. As their parent, you may emotionally and financially support this transition. Colleges, however, cannot legally recognize your involvement without your child's permission. It did always amaze me that the bills for tuition come to parents, but just try and gct information about grades or your child's performance, and the doors are shut pretty tightly.

As a parent, you must decide if you will need access to your child's grades and the ability to interact with the registrar, dean, housing office, or other administrative offices in their college. With my children, I felt that if I was financially responsible for their tuition, then I should be allowed access to the outcome of that investment (i.e., their grades and attendance). I discussed this with them the summer before classes began and reviewed the reasons why I felt it was important for me to have access to that information. They both agreed and were willing to sign FERPA forms. (Fig 5). The FERPA form or Family Educational Rights and Privacy Act allows you, as a parent, the right to access any information listed on the form such as access to their grades and attendance, as well as giving the school and its representatives permission to speak to you about issues that may arise. This form can then be sent to the registrar's office, dean's office, housing office, and the office of disability, if your son or daughter qualifies for those services.

My experience with the medical system following my son's accident also alerted me to the need for a generalized medical release of information form and a power of attorney form. (Figs 6 & 7).

A generalized medical release form allows medical personnel to interact with you if any health issues arise. A power of attorney form allows parents to act in your child's best interest if they are unable to give their consent. A copy of these forms should be kept in your files, as well as on your phone as a photo or PDF in case of an emergency.

Communicating with your college-bound student: A new world awaits your son or daughter as they embark on what may be their first experience living away from home. This will invoke feelings of anxiety in both of you. Some young adults are able to be open and communicative about their anxiety while others are not. Be sensitive as your child draws away from you during the final summer, as they are learning to deal with the mixed feelings of excitement and dread. Being there when they are ready to talk is the best way to allow the avenues of communication to stay open. Allow them to come to you when they are ready. When they are ready to discuss their feelings with you, they will. Forcing the issue will only result in a closed door. Be available, nonjudgmental, and allow them to discuss their feelings on their terms.

Avenues of communication are vitally important during the first six months of college. A few weeks before dropping them off, open a dialogue about how you plan on keeping in touch while they are away. Insisting on some form of communication at least once a week should be acceptable to you both. This can be in the form of text messages, phone calls, or FaceTime or Skype. Ideally, you would want to hear your child's voice or see them via FaceTime or Skype to ascertain how they are coping with their new life. Do they seem engaging and happy to speak to you or are they withdrawn and anxious? Try to ask open-ended questions that allow them to voice their thoughts rather than reply with one-word answers.

Your child's personality should not change drastically during the first several months of college. If you are noticing a significant change, take this as a warning sign. If your child seems to be struggling after several calls, discuss your concerns with them and offer a visit to see them face-to-face. Almost every college student will struggle the first several months, but as a parent, you don't want to miss the warning signs of a child who is becoming increasingly depressed, anxious or isolated.

During your visit, be open with them about your concerns, but most importantly, listen to what they say to you. Be calm, supportive, and ask if they are willing to get help. If you are truly concerned about their mental health, make sure that they are set up with a mental health consultation and follow up to make sure they attended the appointment. If there is a legitimate concern about their immediate mental health, reach out directly to student health services and alert them to the need for immediate intervention.

If you have a freshman, the first time you will see your child on campus is likely parents' visiting day. This may be your first opportunity to ascertain, in person, how well your child is adapting to college. This weekend is a wonderful chance to allow your child to show you their school. If they do not want to attend all of the planned activities, take this as a sign they may just want to spend time with you. Having the opportunity to meet their friends, see their living situation after several months, and perhaps have a meal with them in the cafeteria will help you understand what their day-to-day life is like, and how you might be supportive as they adjust to a new world without your daily presence.

Meeting the resident advisor and college personnel assigned to your child's dorm is another opportunity to connect with those who can be supportive of your child. Save time during the weekend to attend any sessions with your student's academic dean or advisors. They are wonderful resources to help your child adjust to the academic challenges that may lie ahead. If issues arise during the year, do not be hesitant to reach out to those who may help your child, such as a resident advisor or their academic advisor. Believing your student can handle the stress of college is important but reaching out if you feel the need is vitally important.

Drugs/alcohol: Each family will have different views on alcohol use and drug use in your adult child. Several states have transitioned to allowing the legal use of marijuana, and alcohol use on college campus has been prevalent for years. The NIAA reported in a 2015 fact sheet that 1,825 college students between the ages of 18-24 die each year from alcohol related unintentional injuries including motor vehicle accidents. [26]

Alcohol can have a profound affect upon academic performance as well. A 1998 study by Wechsler et al reported that 25% of college students reported alcohol-related academic consequences such as missing class, not being able to keep up with their school work, or performing poorly on tests.[27] A 2009 study showed that students who binge drank (i.e., consumed alcohol more than three times per week) had a significantly higher chance of doing poorly on an exam compared to students who did not binge drink. (40% vs. 7%). This study showed that students who binge drink were much more likely to have missed a class compared to students who did not binge drink (64% vs. 12%).[28]

Certain schools and factors at school have been shown to increase the likelihood of heavy drinking and the consequences that can be associated with this practice. Students who attend schools with a heavy emphasis on Greek life or sports have a higher chance of being exposed to underage drinking. Alcohol consumption is highest among students living in fraternities or sororities and lowest among students who commute to college from home.[29]

These statistics are troubling for any parent, as we all want our children to enjoy that special time in their lives without the dangerous consequences and possible lifelong addiction that can result from the inappropriate use of alcohol. It is important to discuss these issues with your student before they leave for school. What have been your expectations and family rules during high school, and how compliant was your child in following these rules at home? If you have had issues at home, it is likely you will be addressing similar issues at college. A thoughtful discussion about abstinence from alcohol or the thoughtful use of alcohol is the best approach. Start with discussing what your expectations are for responsible alcohol use. Discuss with your child the challenges they may have experienced in high school. Being nonjudgmental and allowing them to discuss their feelings may open the avenues for communication that will be so vital during the first year of college. The NIAAA has an interactive website and College Alcohol Intervention Matirix that can serve as a resource for you and your child to discuss coping strategies for dealing with alcohol exposure at college (www.collegedrinkingprevention.gov/CollegeAIM). Helping your child understand the amount of alcohol that is present in a drink may also help them understand that the practice of pre-gaming, or drinking several drinks in a short amount of time prior to attending an event, can have drastic consequences and lead to alcohol poisoning. (Fig. 8). Discussing the warning signs of alcohol poisoning is also important, so that if a friend or roommate becomes dangerously intoxicated they can respond in an appropriate fashion. (Fig. 9).

It is important to review with your son or daughter their college's website to stress the consequences of underage drinking and how it may affect their college career. For many schools, this information can be found in the academic handbook section of the website. An ongoing discussion about alcohol use and its consequences, as well as your weekly communication, may help you and your child navigate the slippery slope of alcohol abuse.

Mental health issues and your adult child: College can

be a stressful environment for any student, and especially for those with anxiety, depression, eating disorders, or other mental health issues. It is estimated that 20% of the adult population suffers from a mental health disorder.

That number is higher in children 18 to 24 years of age. The Center for Collegiate Mental Health surveyed 93 participating colleges and found that students are making appointments for counseling services at student health-care centers, at a rate of seven times greater than the rate of enrollment (i.e., college enrollment increased 5.6% as compared to an increase of 29.6% in mental health appointments scheduled on college campuses over the past five years). An alarming trend in these national reports was a significant increase in the number of students who considered suicide, from 23.8% in 2010 to 32.9% in 2015. The most common diagnoses treated in this population were anxiety, depression, and social anxiety. These statistics point out an alarming trend in the prevalence of mental health issues among college age young adults.[30]

Communicating with your child about their struggles during the first several months of college is vitally important.

Look for the warning signs that require consultation with a mental health provider:

- Feeling sad or withdrawn for two or more weeks
- Severe, out-of-control risk-taking behaviors

- Sudden overwhelming fears for no reason
- Not eating; throwing up or using laxatives for weight loss
- Seeing, hearing, or believing things that are not real
- Repeated or excessive use of alcohol or drugs
- Drastic changes in: mood, behavior, personality, or sleeping habits
- Extreme difficulty concentrating or staying still
- Intense worries or fears that get in the way of daily activities
- Trying to harm oneself or others

If your child has been diagnosed with a psychiatric disorder prior to leaving home, putting appropriate support services in place prior to their arrival at school is crucial. Assure that they have discussed with their mental health-care provider what types of support they will need. Options are varied and depend upon the student and the severity of their illness.

Continuing Skype or phone sessions with their current provider: The advantage to this option is continuity of care. They hopefully will have made progress with their current health-care provider and this individual knows them and may have a good sense of how to quickly support them as they transition to college. The disadvantage is that the face-to-face interaction is lost and some students may become lax in their weekly sessions.

Finding a mental health provider at college: This option allows for a face-to-face encounter. The therapist at college may also be more familiar with the social life and academic rigors of their college, and can help your child navigate the stressor inherent in independent living in a socially complex and academically challenging environment.

Finding a therapist at college is not always easy. The best resource may be your son's or daughter's current therapist.

If they have worked with a therapist in the area—or with colleagues able to assist in a referral—then you will have a better sense of the quality of the therapist you are helping your child transition to.

Ask your pediatrician if they have worked with therapists near your child's campus, or if they can assist you in researching mental health providers near your child's school. If you are unable to obtain a referral from your current health-care providers, your next step should be to contact student health services at your child's college. They often have a list of therapists they have worked with in the past to help you with your research.

The American Psychiatric Association website has a database of psychiatrists who can be searched by location as well as specialization. The American Psychological Association and *Psychology Today* both have databases on their websites to search psychologists and social workers specializing in mental health by location, specialization, gender, and insurance accepted. Both websites allow clinicians to post personal statements, pictures, and links to their websites, so that you and your student can get a better initial understanding of their treatment philosophy.

Once you have narrowed down your search, your child can set up telephone interviews to help refine their search to one or two therapists. They can then meet with these practitioners at school and decide if the chemistry is right and if they have similar views on how therapy should proceed. If possible, have your child set up appointments with therapists for when you are on campus, so you will have the opportunity to meet with the therapist as well. Ultimately, the decision must be your child's, but most therapists will welcome the opportunity to meet with you early in your child's therapy.

Once a therapeutic alliance has been established, be sure to go over billing, communication, and if the therapist will contact you if your child misses appointments. Your young adult should be a part of this conversation so there are no secrets, and there is a clear understanding between all parties as to how much the therapist can reveal to you regarding your child. Explain to your child that there will be a period of adjustment to the new therapist and that you, their pediatrician, and their former therapist are all resources during the process.

If your child's therapist feels they will need only short-term therapy—or if there are no providers available near your child's college that may be appropriate—obtaining a mental health provider based in the college's psychological services department is an option.Student mental health services will have access to psychiatrists, psychologists and licensed clinical social workers who are all able to provide therapy to your child. It may take longer for your child to make an appointment with the college's mental health services than with a private mental health provider. Students with emergency mental health needs will be given priority.

Although the stigma of mental illness has lessened, ask your child if they have any reservations about utilizing the on-campus mental health services. Being honest with each other up front will help assure that they will feel comfortable with the treatment plan that you and they elect to pursue.

Have your student contact the school to inquire about the number of visits that are available to matriculating students. If you have their permission, you can do it for them. Inquire about the process for choosing a therapist, and ask if changes can be made to the therapeutic assignment if your child does not feel connected to the therapist. Maintain communication between your young adult's current therapist and the school, by having your child submit a medical records release form to student psychological services. The form indicates that reports are to be sent to their primary therapist. (Fig. 10).

There is no way to completely alleviate the anxiety that parents of children with mental health problems experience, especially as they watch their child inch closer to complete independence. Assuring that appropriate support services are in place and keeping an open line of communication with your child will help you trust that they will have a positive experience during their college years.

Chapter 14

Taking Care of Yourself

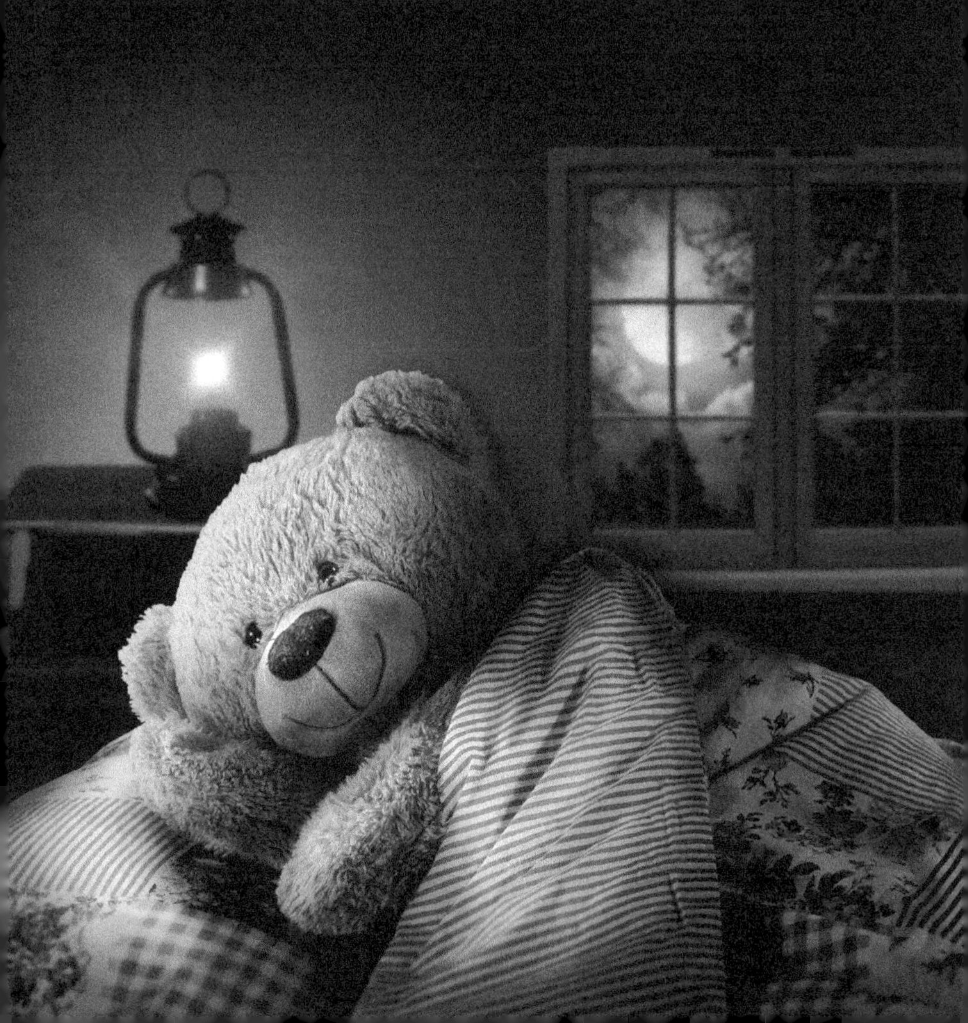

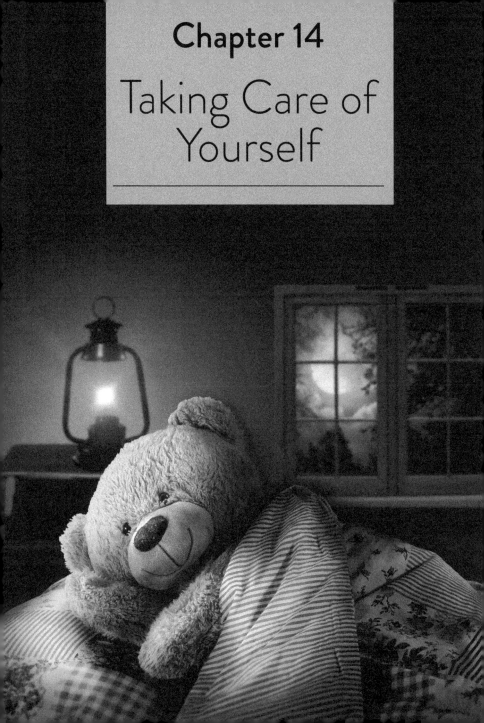

Being a parent is the
hardest job you will ever have.
To be there for your children you must
be there for yourself first.

I hurried to finish the last of my notes of the day and complete all of my outstanding paperwork. I looked down at my desk: the pens were neatly lined up, the outbox full, the inbox empty. I heaved a sigh of relief as I pushed my rather hefty frame away from the desk. A 50-pound weight gain with my second child had left me rather awkward and slow moving. I gathered my coat and waved to the janitor as I headed to the elevator.

"Good luck tomorrow," he called.

I wasn't sure luck had much to do with my upcoming delivery but I smiled as I walked by and headed to the door.

I was so happy the day would finally be upon me to shed the extra weight I had been lugging around in the hot, humid heat of the New York City summer. I had the next several weeks planned to the hour. I would deliver my baby, rest for a few days, and then drive out to Eastern Long Island to spend the remainder of August in the cool breezes of Long Island Sound. I had signed up my older son for day camp and the baby and I would relax on the lawn and have a chance to get to know each other.

My delivery was harrowing for both the obstetrician and me. An emergency C-section had ruined our plans for a calm, controlled delivery, but all of us had survived with my obstetrician telling me that another pregnancy on my part might be the end of our friendship. My husband wheeled our infant son and me across the street to our apartment where I rested overnight and insisted he ready the car with our belongings.

Six years of marriage had taught my husband that when my mind was made up, it was just easier to go with the flow and he piled the children, our cats, and me into the car and began the long drive east.

My first few days were blissful. My husband entertained our older son and the baby—still in the stupor of delivery, was sleepy and calm. Sunday night arrived and my husband reached for my hand."Are you sure you will be okay alone with the kids?" he asked.

"Of course, I will!" I confidently replied.

I worked 12 hours a day, 6 days a week. This would be a vacation.

He climbed into the car and I watched as his headlights disappeared into the inky blackness of the quiet country road.

The shrill wail of my infant son woke me at 5 a.m. I fed and changed him as the red glow of the rising summer sun crept across the floor of my bedroom. I readied my older son's lunch and his clothes and gently kissed his tousled curls as he lay sleeping.

"Time to get up my love," I gently caressed his shoulder as he turned towards me, his deep brown eyes flickering open.

"It's time to get ready for camp," I murmured. He abruptly sat up in bed, his five-year-old face set in a frown.

"I'm not going to camp, I'm staying here with you," he said.

"No, no, camp will be wonderful," I replied.

"No, Mom, camp is stupid, I'll just stay here," I led him downstairs and made a bowl of cereal. As the hands of the clock moved closer to 8:30 a.m., I tempted him outside with a ball and glove. Thank goodness the baby lay peacefully sleeping in his bassinet by the front door. As we threw the ball back and forth, the camp bus pulled into the driveway. The door swung open and an energetic teenager bounded down the stairs.

"Hi, I'm Emily. Would you like to come meet some new friends?"

His face went blank and he looked from me to the bus and dropped to the ground with his face buried in his hands."No camp, Mom, I'm not going." he said. Emily and I tried every trick to engage him, but my strong-willed son was not budging.

Finally, Emily shrugged her shoulders, smiled, and bounded back on the bus.

"Give us a call if he changes his mind," she waved, and the bus backed noisily out of my driveway.

The next several days were a blur of chicken nuggets and dirty diapers. Thank goodness for the "Teenage Mutant Ninja Turtles." My son watched hours and hours of TV as I attempted to move from one task to the other.

How could this be so hard? I felt inadequate and overwhelmed. By the end of the week, I was exhausted and feeling sick. My husband arrived and I collapsed into the bed.

At 3 a.m., I awoke shivering and covered in sweat.

"John, I'm really not feeling well. I feel hot," I said.

"No, you're fine," he murmured, laying his hand on my arm. "Go back to sleep. I'll give the baby a bottle."

By morning, I could hardly move and there was a sharp pain in my abdomen. I shook my husband awake.

"Get the kids and the car, we are going home."

The drive home felt as if it took hours. The sweat dripped from my brow and I struggled to get comfortable. I paged my obstetrician who met me at the emergency room. The next several days were spent in a stupor of sleep and medication.

I received IV antibiotics and pain medication to treat the infection that had developed after my C-section. As my fever slowly dissipated, I lay in the hospital bed realizing that I could not do this alone. It was just too hard. I picked up the phone and reached out for help, and it arrived within hours. My husband, my friends, my family, and my colleagues all pitched in to help over the next several weeks. It was hard for me to admit that I could not do it alone—but I couldn't, and that realization was liberating.

Being a parent is the hardest job you will ever have. You will give up your freedom, your resources, and in some instances, your sanity. To be there for your children you must be there for yourself first. Learning how to nourish your spirit can only help you to nourish theirs.

Your health: Learning to care for yourself is of vital importance. Eating correctly, getting exercise, and trying to manage stress will have long-term benefits to keeping you healthy as your child matures and grows.

It is tempting to eat chicken nuggets from your son's plate, or fill the refrigerator with ice cream and snacks for your teenage son, but refrain from making those items a staple in your diet. Your child learns eating habits from you, so concentrating on a well-balanced diet is as important for your child as it is for you. Keep coffee, alcohol, and sugar to a minimum, especially during the stages in your child's development when your sleep cycle needs to mirror theirs (i.e., during the first few years of life, and during the teenage years when the hours until they walk in the door with the car keys seem never-ending).

Exercise is a critical part of your health-care plan. Regular exercise helps combat stress, tones your muscles, and helps you shed the excess weight of pregnancy. A jump rope and weights make a wonderful bedside gym and can be used as soon as you are cleared by your OB to start exercising again.

Many local gyms have babysitting facilities and this is a great way to meet other parents who are coping with the same issues that you face. Coordinate with your spouse or partner a way that you can both have alone time to keep fit. Setting a schedule and attempting to stick with it will give both of you the opportunity to concentrate on getting stronger and maintaining your health.

As your child grows, you can share sports together such as basketball, bike riding, tennis, or skiing—spending time together engaged in physical activity is beneficial to your relationship and your health. Signing up for swimming class together is a great way to bond and have quality time together while exercising.

Planning one family vacation per year that is active will set a framework for how you and your children relax together. Camping, hiking, or canoeing are wonderful activities to share together. Ski trips or bike trips—whether they are close to home or across the country—will make memories your children will treasure forever. If your family is not the active type, set realistic expectations on what you can achieve together. Relaxation, fun, and time spent together are the most important aspects to concentrate on.

Managing your stress is also an important life lesson for any parent. It seems the stress of raising your newborn infant can be overwhelming until you experience the special brand of stress reserved for the parents of teenagers.

The mantra, "little kids, little problems; big kids, big problems" never seemed so true as you watch your child navigate the minefield of young adulthood.

Learn early on what helps you deal with the stress of everyday life and what you can do to establish a routine that allows you to be proactive in addressing your stress.

Stress can be contagious. Our children can pick up on the stress we project and internalize it. This is thought to occur through mirror neurons. Mirror neurons are brain cells that react in a similar way to performing an act or observing an act. These neurons are also thought to be able to perceive the intent behind an action. That intent and its action are mirrored in the brain causing neurons in the observer's brain to fire.[31]

These neurons were first discovered in the brains of monkeys.

Studies in humans have shown that we have similar brain activity. Humans researchers have termed our ability to learn through watching other's behavior, observational learning.[32] This can be seen in the smile mirrored by newborn babies when we smile at them. Authors postulate that negative emotions and behavior can also be mirrored in our children. If we project frequent anxiety, stress, or depression, the mirror neurons in our children may start to internalize these behaviors. This research confirms how important it is to take care of ourselves so that we can raise happy, healthy, and well-adapted children.

What are some of the strategies we can utilize to de-stress?

Unplug: Constantly checking your email, Facebook, or texts sends a message to your children that you are not there "in the moment" with them. We are all guilty of sneaking a peek at work email while supposedly relaxing at home. Set a time where no one is connected to the outside world—no computers and no cell phones. Whether this is playtime with small children or dinnertime with your teens, be present, be focused on them, and let the outside world wait.

Mindfulness: Incorporating stress reduction practices into your daily life can take just a few minutes a day. Whether it is meditation, deep breathing or yoga, these are all strategies that both you and your children can add to your daily routine. Imagine sitting on the bed each night with your five-year-old child, and learning the art of clearing your mind and relaxing for five minutes. By the time they are 16 and the unavoidable stress of high school occurs, they will have mastered techniques to keep them grounded, and calm themselves.

Make time for self-care: Whether it is taking a nightly bath with a good magazine, reading a good book (my favorite!) or getting a massage or facial, make time for things that make you feel good. The hour you spend away from your children concentrating on yourself will make the hours you spend with them more enjoyable for you both, as you will be more relaxed and focused on them.

Don't neglect your friends: Spending time with friends is a wonderful way to concentrate on yourself. Research has shown that friendships suffer during parenthood. A study of 1,000 parents showed that prior to having children, men spent 16 hours a week with friends, and after having children they spent only 6 hours. Prior to motherhood, participants in the study reported spending 14 hours a week with friends, and after delivery they spent only 5 hours.

What you rely on your friends for during parenthood may also change. Before having children, 90% of women relied on their friends for fun, but after having children this number dropped to 50%, with 56% feeling that having friends who were good listeners was more important.[33]

Avoid negative people, and fill your life with friends who

have positive outlooks and can be there for you if you call (and do call!). Cultivating relationships with parents of your children's classmates has the added advantage of building a support network for both you and your child. Modeling healthy relationships with your peers will help your children understand how to be a good friend and the benefits of healthy relationships with others.

Make your spouse as important in your life as your children: This is a difficult task, as being a parent can, for many of us, be all-encompassing. Your children become the center of your life and your spouse quickly falls to number two. Linda and Charles Bloom in their book, *101 Things I Wish I Knew When I Got Married: Simple Lessons to Make Love Last*, says that when couples make the needs of their children paramount in the home, their relationship with their spouse can suffer.

This can lead to feelings of anger, resentment, loneliness, and frustration on the part of one or both participants in the marriage.[34]

Children want to feel loved and appreciated, but constant attention and focus on their every action and mood makes it more difficult for them to grow up to be self-reliant, confident adults. They also observe that marriage is not an enjoyable place to be. How can you be a great parent and a great spouse at the same time? Set aside time for both.

We all have mealtime and bedtime rituals with our children—eating dinner together or reading a book. Set up rituals to concentrate on your marriage. Arrange for weekly or biweekly date nights with your spouse. Hire a babysitter or rotate childcare with a friend or relative. The amount you spend on a babysitter several times per month will pale in comparison to the amount you will spend on legal fees for your divorce!

Communicate with your spouse. Tell them you love them, and mean it. Leave notes in their purse, briefcase, or lunch bag. Anything that shows you are thinking of them, and them alone. Try and go away together once or twice a year. This does not have to be an exotic or expensive trip; you can even send the children to a friend's or relative's house for the weekend. Reconnect, relax, and spend the days just concentrating on each other and remembering why you married that person in the first place.

Make sex a priority in your marriage. Find ways to connect on both an emotional and physical level. If you're finding you're just too exhausted to be physical with your partner, finds ways to relax such as massages or baths together. Show your partner that the physical act of expressing your love and commitment to each other is an important part of your life. Both of you will benefit from it.

The safety instructions that we hear on the plane are important to remember:

"Put your oxygen mask on first, before you help others."

Your health—both mental and physical—will make you a more caring and competent parent.

Chapter 15
Conclusion

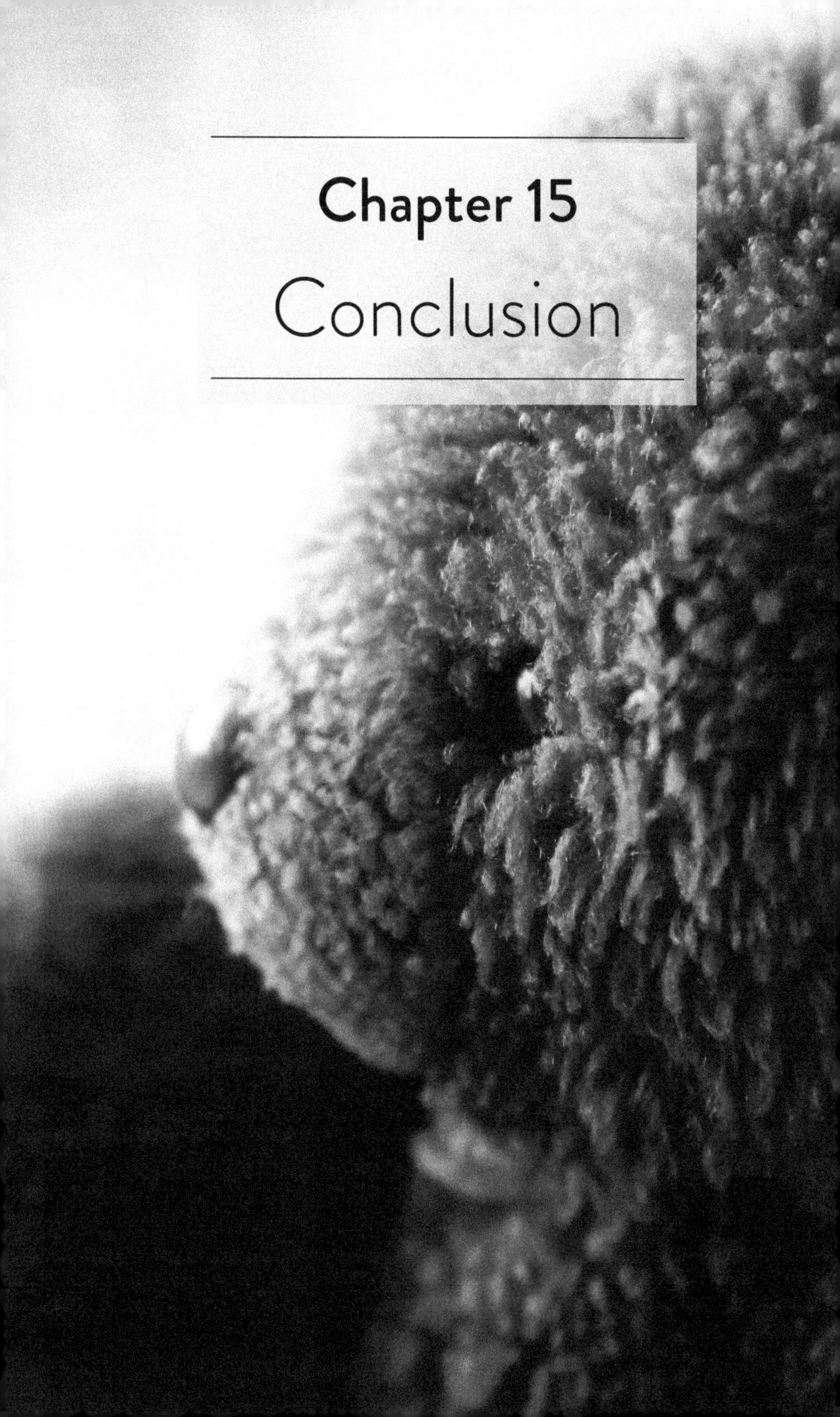

As a mother, I could not give up wanting the best for my child. I wanted him to be safe and comfortable, loved and protected.

I couldn't help myself. My shopping cart was almost filled as I wheeled around the California Walmart getting what I believed were essentials for my second child's dorm room. It was his first time living away from home for an extended period, and I was intent on making him comfortable. A table light, comfy sheets, new pillows, a wastepaper basket (oh, and look at that great rug!)—item after item filled my cart. I knew I shouldn't be doing this. I had learned so much from my first son as he transitioned to college. Trust that they will make the right decisions, give them space to grow and make their own mistakes, be there for them when they need you but don't overstay your welcome. I knew all these things in my heart, but if his bed was uncomfortable or his feet were cold at night, he would appreciate my efforts then. As I wheeled my cart around the corner, my six-foot-tall son stood at the end of the aisle staring at me.

"No, Mom. Just put it back. I don't need any of it."

"But sweetie, your pillows are old and that comforter you brought is from middle school. This will be so much nicer," I pleaded.

"Nope. Mom, just put it back. I'll be fine."

I followed him to the checkout where I paid for the toothpaste, deodorant, and face cream he had bought. Experience had taught me that arguing at this point was futile and I reluctantly followed him out to the car.

When we arrived at his dorm room, my resourceful husband had accomplished the most important tasks of hooking up the TV and attaching the requisite wall hanging over his bed. He dropped his supplies in the bathroom and looked me steadily in the eye.

"Guess it's time for you to go," he smiled, and looked towards the door.

"Are you sure you don't want to join us for dinner? We're staying just down the road." Anything to have a few more minutes with him before I relinquished him to adulthood."Nope. Mom. it's time to leave. I'll see you in October. You're coming back for parents' visiting day, remember?"

"Yes, of course. Let me check to make sure your bed is made."

"No, Mom, it's fine." He walked forward and embraced me, my head landing just in the middle of his chest. I held on tight and gave him a hug that I hoped would last the eight weeks until I saw him again.

"Love you sweetie," I murmured and stepped away.

He walked us to the door and I promised myself I would not cry. When I dropped my firstborn off at college, I sobbed the whole way home. I considered my self-control, at this point, a true victory. As my husband held my hand and I walked slowly away from my boy, I pondered how much had changed in these past five years and how much had stayed the same. As a mother, I could not give up wanting the best for my child. I wanted him to be safe and comfortable, loved and protected. That would never change. I had, however, grown and matured as a parent. I knew when it was time to let him have his own experiences, both positive and negative, for that is how our children grow to be responsible adults. As hard as it might be to let go, that is what I needed to do. As I sat in the car feeling the warm California breeze on my face, I let my tears fall. I knew what I needed to do and I had done it. That didn't make the pain of leaving him any easier, for that is what being a parent means. Loving your children to distraction, but letting them go when the time arrives and trusting that both you, and they, will continue to grow and mature.

I hope this book has brought you insight into the complicated, messy, and indescribably wonderful world of parenting. As a mother and a physician, I shared my personal stories with you in the hope that they have helped you to understand how deeply I care for my children—both those I have born, and those who I care for with their parents.By being an active engaged participant in your child's care, they will receive the optimum experience that both you and their physician want them to receive. Please remember that as physicians, we want to be partners in your child's care. You, as a parent, are a vital and important part of that health care alliance.

Please stay connected through the frequent blogs on my website, jacquelinejonesent.com, as well as updates and useful articles on my Twitter and Facebook pages. For those of you who live in New York City and the surrounding area, I welcome you to join my family of patients. Please visit my website to book appointments or contact me. I look forward to keeping in touch.

Figure 1

Category	Medical Assistant	Nurse (RN, BSN)	Nurse Practitioner	Physician Assistant	Physician (Family Practice)
Prerequisite Education	None	None	Bachelor Degree in Nursing and clinical hours	Bachelor Degree and clinical hours	Bachelor Degree
Learning Model	-	Medical-Nursing	Medical-Nursing	Medical-Physician	Medical-Physician
Time in Classroom	134 hrs	varies greatly by program	500 hrs	1000 hrs	2 years
Time in Clinic	160 hours	varies by program	500-700 hrs	2000 hrs	2 years
Total Post High School Education	1-2 years	2-4 years	6-8 years	6-7 years	8 years
Residency	None	None	None	Optional 1-2 years	3-8 years
Degree or Certificate Awarded	Certificate or Associate Degree	Associate or Bachelor Degree	Master's Degree planned transition to Doctorate	Master's Degree PA-C	Doctor of Medicine (M.D.) or Osteopathy (D.O.)
Recertification	60 education points or exam every 5 years	1000 hours practicing in area of certification or exam every 5 years	1000 professional practice hours and 12 CE credits per year OR exam every 5 years	100 education hours every 2 years and exam every 10 years	MD: 50 education hours/year and ABMS certification recommended
Base Salary U.S	$29,708	$66,220 (varies greatly by state)	$97,990	$97,280	$185,151
Independent Practitioner			18 states allow NPs to practice independently		Yes
Complicated or High Risk Cases			Varies	Varies	Yes
Perform Surgery			Assist	Assist	Yes
Deliver babies			Yes	Varies by State	Yes
Write Prescriptions			Yes	Yes	Yes
Prescribe Controlled Substances			Varies by State	Varies by State	Yes
Conduct Physical Exams		Assist	Yes	Yes	Yes
Diagnose			Yes	Yes	Yes
Treat Illness		Yes	Yes	Yes	Yes
Order and Interpret Tests		Assist	Yes	Yes	Yes
Patient [illegible]		Yes	Yes	Yes	Yes

Figure 2

Oral Health During Pregnancy

- Brush your teeth gently twice a day with a soft bristled toothbrush and a toothpaste containing fluoride. Your toothbrush should easily fit inside your mouth allowing you to reach all areas within your mouth easily.

- Replace your toothbrush every three or four months or sooner if the bristles are worn or frayed. A worn toothbrush won't do a good job of cleaning your teeth and can cause irritate of your gums.

- Clean between your teeth with floss or another interdental cleaner each day. This process helps remove the plaque that forms on your teeth and under the gum line which can lead to gingivitis and increase your chances of bleeding from your gums during pregnancy.

- Eat a healthy diet made up of various foods from the following groups:
  Grains
  Vegetables
  Fruits
  Diary Products
  Protein
  Fats or Oils

- Try to limit your snacking. When you consume foods or beverages that contain sugar the bacterial in your mouth release acid that attack your teeth, increasing your chance of developing cavities.

- Visit your dentist early in your pregnancy and advise both your obstetrician and dentist or any issues that arise with your oral health.

- For further information about your oral health during pregnancy visit the American Dental Association website (www.ada. org) or consult your dentist.

Adapted from the American Dental Association. Keeping your mouth healthy during pregnancy. *JADA.2013;144(11).* http://jada.ada.org.1314

Figure 3

Baby Teeth Eruption Chart

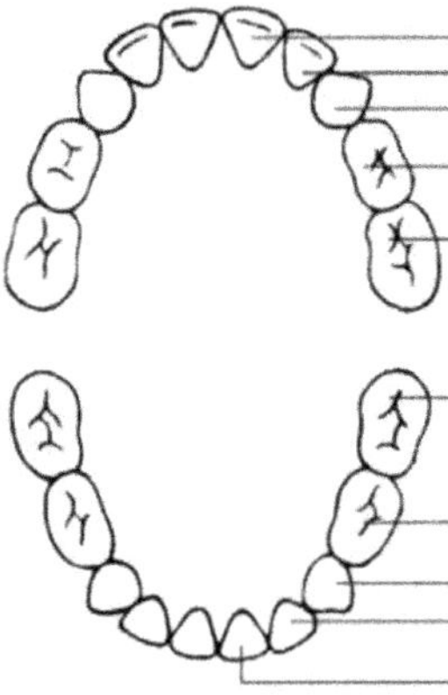

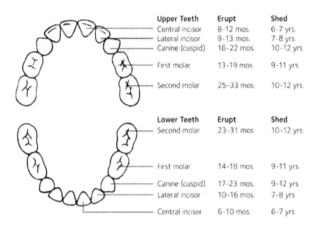

Upper Teeth	Erupt	Shed
Central incisor	8-12 mos.	6-7 yrs.
Lateral incisor	9-13 mos.	7-8 yrs.
Canine (cuspid)	16-22 mos.	10-12 yrs.
First molar	13-19 mos.	9-11 yrs.
Second molar	25-33 mos.	10-12 yrs.

Lower Teeth	Erupt	Shed
Second molar	23-31 mos.	10-12 yrs.
First molar	14-18 mos.	9-11 yrs.
Canine (cuspid)	17-23 mos.	9-12 yrs.
Lateral incisor	10-16 mos.	7-8 yrs.
Central incisor	6-10 mos.	6-7 yrs.

Permanent Teeth Eruption Chart

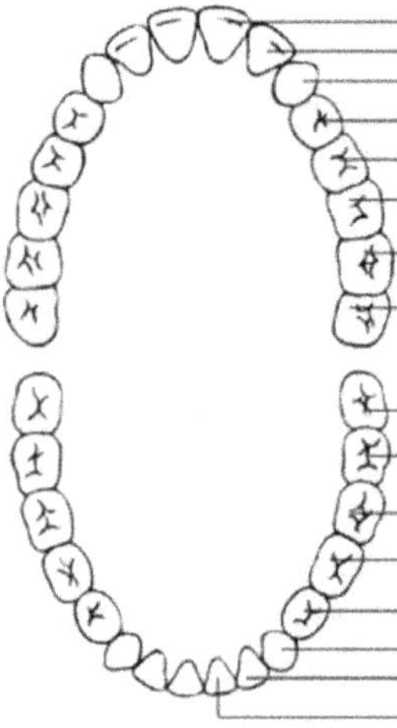

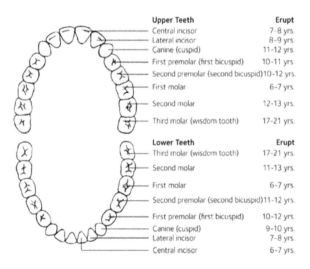

Upper Teeth	Erupt
Central incisor	7-8 yrs.
Lateral incisor	8-9 yrs.
Canine (cuspid)	11-12 yrs.
First premolar (first bicuspid)	10-11 yrs.
Second premolar (second bicuspid)	10-12 yrs.
First molar	6-7 yrs.
Second molar	12-13 yrs.
Third molar (wisdom tooth)	17-21 yrs.

Lower Teeth	Erupt
Third molar (wisdom tooth)	17-21 yrs.
Second molar	11-13 yrs.
First molar	6-7 yrs.
Second premolar (second bicuspid)	11-12 yrs.
First premolar (first bicuspid)	10-12 yrs.
Canine (cuspid)	9-10 yrs.
Lateral incisor	7-8 yrs.
Central incisor	6-7 yrs.

Figure 4

AUTHORIZATION FOR RELEASE OF MEDICAL INFORMATION
TO PARENTS OR GUARDIANS

Patient's Name: ______________________

Patient's Date of Birth: ______________________

I authorize (Physician) to release my medical information solely to my parents or guardians:

Parents or Guardians Name: ______________________

Address: ______________________

Phone Number: ______________________

This authorization is valid until revoked.

I understand that the disclosure of this health information is voluntary. I can refuse to sign this authorization.

I further understand that any disclosure of information carries with it the potential for an unauthorized re-disclosure and the information may not be protected by federal privacy regulations. If I have questions about disclosures of health care, I may contact (Physician) or the Practice Administrator.

I have the right to revoke this authorization in writing at any time.

______________________ ______________________

Patient Signature Date

Figure 5

Disclosure to Parents of Dependent Students and Consent Form for Disclosure to Parents

To: Registrar
[Postsecondary Institution]

From: ____

Student's First Name   Middle Initial   Last Name

____

Permanent Street Address   City   State   Zip Code

Under the Family Educational Rights and Privacy Act (FERPA), the [**Postsecondary Institution**] is permitted to disclose information from your education records to your parents if your parents (or one of your parents) claim you as a dependent for federal tax purposes. Please indicate whether your parents claim you as a tax dependent.

Please check the appropriate box:

☐ Yes. I certify that my parents claim me as a dependent for federal income tax purposes.

☐ No. I certify that my parents do not claim me as a dependent for federal income tax purposes.

Signature: ______________________ **Date**: ______________________

If you are not claimed as a dependent or you do not know whether you are claimed as a dependent for federal income tax purposes, but you agree that [**Postsecondary Institution**] may disclose information from your education records to your parents, please sign the following consent:

I consent to the dislosure of any personally identitifiable information from my education records to my parent(s), for reasons determined by the [Postsecondary Institution] as appropriate. This authorization will remain in effect for the (current year) school year.

Signature: ______________________ **Date**: ______________________

If parents live at the same address, please list both in # 1.

1. Name(s) ______________________

   Address ______________________

   City, State, Zip ______________________

   Telephone ______________________

2. Name(s) ______________________

   Address ______________________

   City, State, Zip ______________________

   Telephone ______________________

Figure 5

What is *FERPA*?

The *Family Educational Rights and Privacy Act* (*FERPA*) is a federal privacy law that gives parents certain protections with regard to their children's education records, such as report cards, transcripts, disciplinary records, contact and family information, and class schedules. As a parent, you have the right to review your child's education records and to request changes under limited circumstances. To protect your child's privacy, the law generally requires schools to ask for written consent before disclosing your child's personally identifiable information to individuals other than you.

The following questions and answers are intended to help you understand your rights as a parent under *FERPA*. If you have further questions, please contact the U.S. Department of Education's Family Policy Compliance Office using the contact information provided below.

My child's school won't show me her or his education records. Does the school have to provide me with a copy of the records if I request them?

Schools must honor your request to review your child's education records within 45 days of receiving the request. Some states have laws similar to *FERPA* that require schools to provide access within a shorter period of time. *FERPA* requires that schools provide parents with an opportunity to inspect and review education records, but not to receive copies, except in limited circumstances.

Parents whose children receive services under the *Individuals with Disabilities Education Act* (*IDEA*) may have additional rights and remedies with regard to their children's education records. The school district, local special education director, or state special education director can answer questions about *IDEA*.

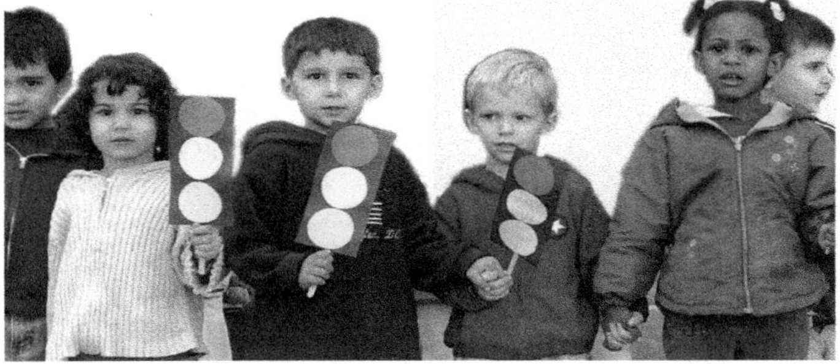

Who else gets to see my child's education records?

To protect your child's privacy, schools are generally prohibited from disclosing personally identifiable information about your child without your written consent. Exceptions to this rule include:

- disclosures made to school officials with legitimate educational interests;
- disclosures made to another school at which the student intends to enroll;
- disclosures made to state or local education authorities for auditing or evaluating federal- or state-supported education programs, or enforcing federal laws that relate to those programs; and
- disclosures including information the school has designated as "directory information."

What is directory information?

FERPA defines "directory information" as information contained in a student's education record that generally would not be considered harmful or an invasion of privacy if disclosed. Directory information could include:

- name, address, telephone listing, electronic mail address, date and place of birth, dates of attendance, and grade level;
- participation in officially recognized activities and sports;
- weight and height of members of athletic teams;
- degrees, honors, and awards received; and
- the most recent school attended.

Figure 5

A school may disclose directory information to anyone, without consent, if it has given parents: general notice of the information it has designated as "directory information"; the right to opt out of these disclosures; and the period of time they have to notify the school of their desire to opt out.

Does *FERPA* give me a right to see the education records of my son or daughter who is in college?

When a student turns 18 years old or enters a postsecondary institution at any age, all rights afforded to you as a parent under *FERPA* transfer to the student ("eligible student"). However, *FERPA* provides ways in which a school may—but is not required to—share information from an eligible student's education records with parents, without the student's consent. For example:

- Schools may disclose education records to parents if the student is claimed as a dependent for tax purposes.
- Schools may disclose education records to parents if a health or safety emergency involves their son or daughter.
- Schools may inform parents if the student, if he or she is under age 21, has violated any law or policy concerning the use or possession of alcohol or a controlled substance.
- A school official may generally share with a parent information that is based on that official's personal knowledge or observation of the student.

Contact Information

For further information about *FERPA*, contact the Department's Family Policy Compliance Office.

Family Policy Compliance Office
U.S. Department of Education
400 Maryland Ave. S.W.
Washington, DC 20202-5920
202-260-3887

For quick, informal responses to routine questions about *FERPA*, parents may also e-mail the Family Policy Compliance Office at *FERPA.Customer@ED.Gov*.

Additional information and guidance may be found at FPCO's Web site at: http://www.ed.gov/policy/gen/guid/fpco/index.html.

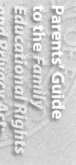

Parents' Guide to the *Family Educational Rights and Privacy Act*: Rights Regarding Children's Education Records

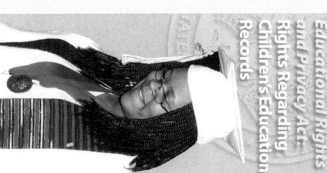

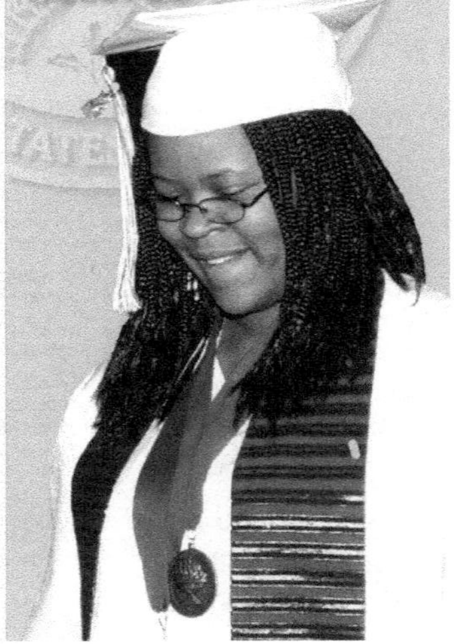

Figure 6

Medical Release of Information/HIPAA Privacy Authorization Form

Authorization for Use or Disclosure of Protected Health Information (Required by the Health Insurance Portability and Accountability Act, 45 C.F.R. Parts 160 and 164)

1. Authorization

I authorize ______________________________(healthcare provider) to use and disclose the protected health information described below to

______________________(individual seeking the information).

2. Effective Period

This authorization for release of information covers the period of healthcare from:

a. ☐ _____________ to _____________

.

OR

b. ☐ All past, present and future periods.

3. Extent of Authorization

a. ☐ I authorize the release of my complete health record (including records relating to mental healthcare, communicable diseases, HIV or AIDS, and treatment of alcohol or drug abuse).

Figure 6

Medical Release of Information/HIPAA Privacy Authorization Form

Authorization for Use or Disclosure of Protected Health Information (Required by the Health Insurance Portability and Accountability Act, 45 C.F.R. Parts 160 and 164)

1. Authorization

I authorize ______________________________(healthcare provider) to use and disclose the protected health information described below to ______________________(individual seeking the information).

2. Effective Period

This authorization for release of information covers the period of healthcare from:

a. □ ____________ to ____________.

OR

b. □ All past, present and future periods.

3. Extent of Authorization

a. □ I authorize the release of my complete health record (including records relating to mental healthcare, communicable diseases, HIV or AIDS, and treatment of alcohol or drug abuse).

OR

b. □ I authorize the release of my complete health record with the exception of the following information:
□ Mental health records
□ Communicable diseases (including HIV and AIDS)
□ Alcohol/drug abuse treatment

Figure 7

DURABLE POWER OF ATTORNEY

Should include, at the minimum, the following elements. Consult an attorney or obtain state specific forms by searching " Free power of attorney forms for ____________(state)". Forms should be valid for both the state where you reside and the states where your child will attend college. Information on health care proxy forms for a specific state can be obtained by visiting www.caringinfo.org or searching " Health Care Proxy forms for _______(state)".

1. Nature of Power- Financial and Health Care Proxy

2. Agent- Preferable parent but a trusted adult can be named

3. Effective Date- immediately

4. Powers of Agent- Should include but are not limited to:

- **Management of Personal Property**
- **Real Estate Transactions**
- **Banking Transactions**
- **Insurance Transactions**
- **Claims and Litigation Matters**
- **Tax Matters**
- **Government Benefits**
- **Employ Required Professionals**

8. Nomination of Guardian or Conservator

Figure 8

Amount of Alcohol in a Drink

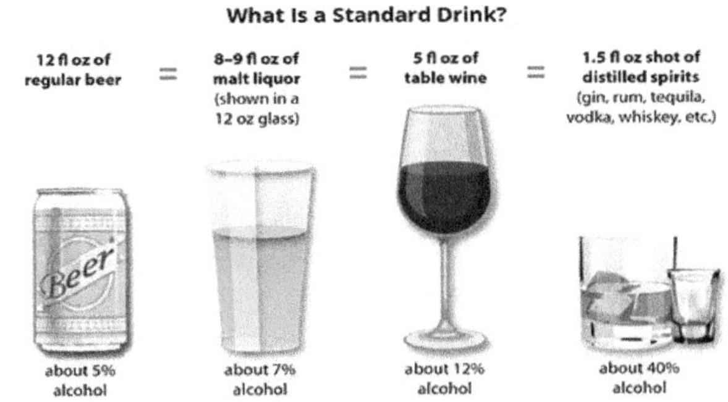

Each beverage portrayed above represents one standard drink of "pure" alcohol, defined in the United States as 0.6 fl oz or 14 grams. The percent of pure alcohol, expressed here as alcohol by volume (alc/vol), varies within and across beverage types. Although the standard drink amounts are helpful for following health guidelines, they may not reflect customary serving sizes.

National Institute on Alcoholism and Alcohol Abuse:
Understanding the impact of alcohol on human health and well-being
www.niaaa.nih.gov

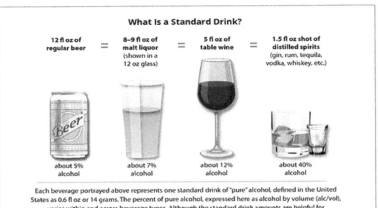

Figure 9

National Institute
on Alcohol Abuse
and Alcoholism

Alcohol Overdose: The Dangers of Drinking Too Much

Celebrating at parties, cheering a favorite sports team, and simply enjoying a break from work are common activities throughout the year. For some people, these occasions also may include drinking—even drinking to excess. And the results can be deadly.

Although many people enjoy moderate drinking, defined as 1 drink per day for women or 2 for men, drinking too much can lead to an overdose. An overdose of alcohol occurs when a person has a blood alcohol content (or BAC) sufficient to produce impairments that increase the risk of harm. Overdoses can range in severity, from problems with balance and slurred speech to coma or even death. What tips the balance from drinking that has pleasant effects to drinking that can cause harm varies among individuals. Age, drinking experience, gender, the amount of food eaten, even ethnicity all can influence how much is too much.

Underage drinkers may be at particular risk for alcohol overdose. Research shows that people under age 20 typically drink about 5 drinks at one time.[1] Drinking such a large quantity of alcohol can overwhelm the body's ability to break down and clear alcohol from the bloodstream. This leads to rapid increases in BAC and significantly impairs brain function.

As BAC increases, so do alcohol's effects—as well as the risk for harm. Even small increases in BAC can decrease coordination, make a person feel sick, and cloud judgment. This can lead to injury from falls or car crashes, leave one vulnerable to sexual assault or other acts of violence, and increase

Critical Signs and Symptoms of Alcohol Poisoning

- Mental confusion, stupor, coma, or inability to wake up
- Vomiting
- Seizures
- Slow breathing (fewer than 8 breaths per minute)
- Irregular breathing (10 seconds or more between breaths)
- Hypothermia (low body temperature), bluish skin color, paleness

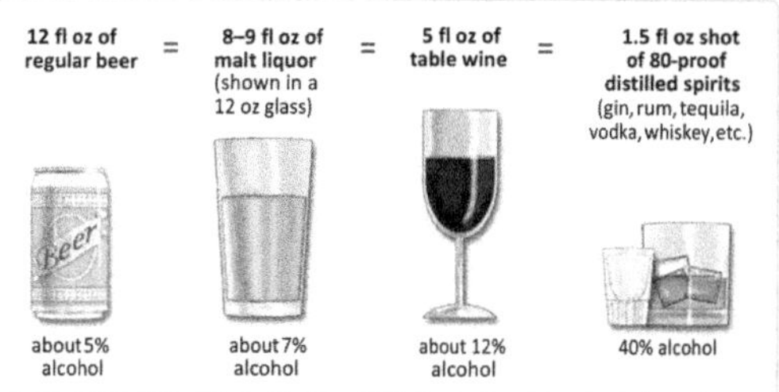

The percent of "pure" alcohol, expressed here as alcohol by volume (alc/vol), varies by beverage.

Although the "standard" drink amounts are helpful for following health guidelines, they may not reflect customary serving sizes. In addition, while the alcohol concentrations listed are "typical," there is considerable variability in alcohol content within each type of beverage (e.g., beer, wine, distilled spirits).

Figure 9

BAC can continue to rise even when a person stops drinking or is unconscious. Alcohol in the stomach and intestine continues to enter the bloodstream and circulate throughout the body.

It is dangerous to assume that an unconscious person will be fine by sleeping it off. One potential danger of alcohol overdose is choking on one's own vomit. Alcohol at very high levels can hinder signals in the brain that control automatic responses such as the gag reflex. With no gag reflex, a person who drinks to the point of passing out is in danger of choking on his or her vomit and dying from a lack of oxygen (i.e., asphyxiation). Even if the person survives, an alcohol overdose like this can lead to long-lasting brain damage.

Know the Danger Signs and Act Quickly

Know the danger signals and, if you suspect that someone has an alcohol overdose, call 911 for help immediately. Do not wait for the person to have all the symptoms, and be aware that a person who has passed out can die. Don't play doctor—cold showers, hot coffee, and walking do not reverse the effects of alcohol overdose and could actually make things worse.

While waiting for medical help to arrive:

- Be prepared to provide information to the responders, including the type and amount of alcohol the person drank; other drugs he or she took, if known; and any health information that you know about the person, such as medications currently taking, allergies to medications, and any existing health conditions.
- Do not leave an intoxicated person alone, as he or she is at risk of getting injured from falling or choking. Keep the person on the ground in a sitting or partially upright position rather than in a chair.
- Help a person who is vomiting. Have him or her lean forward to prevent choking. If a person is unconscious or lying down, roll him or her onto one side with an ear toward the ground to prevent choking.

Stay alert to keep your friends and family safe. And remember—you can avoid the risk of an alcohol overdose by drinking responsibly if you choose to drink, or by not drinking at all.

Critical Signs and Symptoms of an Alcohol Overdose

- Mental confusion, stupor
- Difficulty remaining conscious, or inability to wake up
- Vomiting
- Seizures
- Slow breathing (fewer than 8 breaths per minute)
- Irregular breathing (10 seconds or more between breaths)
- Slow heart rate
- Clammy skin
- Dulled responses, such as no gag reflex (which prevents choking)
- Extremely low body temperature, bluish skin color, or paleness

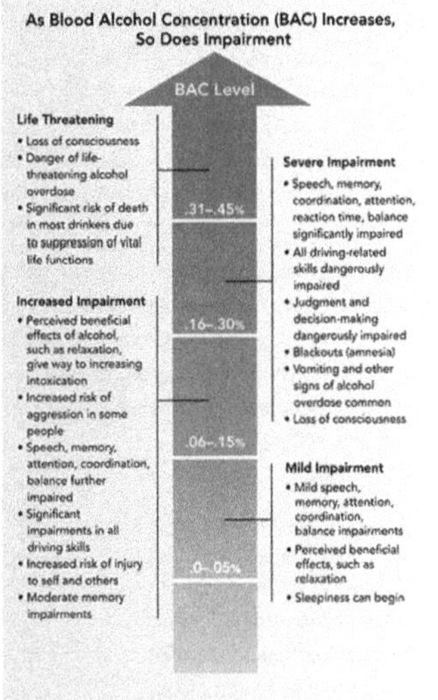

Please note that the BAC ranges depicted in this graph are not absolute and vary by individual.

For more information, please visit: **https://www.niaaa.nih.gov**

[1]National Institute on Alcohol Abuse and Alcoholism. NIAAA Council approves definition of binge drinking. *NIAAA Newsletter*, No. 3, Winter 2004. https://pubs.niaaa.nih.gov/publications/Newsletter/winter2004/Newsletter_Number3.pdf. Accessed September 5, 2018.

[2] Hingson, R.W.; Zha, W.; and White, A.M. Drinking beyond the binge threshold: Predictors, consequences, and changes in the U.S. *American Journal of Preventive Medicine* 52(6):717–727, 2017. PMID: 28526355

Updated October 2018

Figure 9

Alcohol also can irritate the stomach, causing vomiting. With no gag reflex, a person who drinks to the point of passing out is in danger of choking on vomit, which, in turn, could lead to death by asphyxiation. Even if the drinker survives, an alcohol overdose can lead to long-lasting brain damage.

If you suspect someone has alcohol poisoning, get medical help immediately. Cold showers, hot coffee, or walking will not reverse the effects of alcohol overdose and could actually make things worse.

At the hospital, medical staff will manage any breathingproblems, administer fluids to combat dehydration and low blood sugar, and flush the drinker's stomach to help clear the body of toxins.

The best way to avoid an alcohol overdose is to drink responsibly if you choose to drink.

According to the Dietary Guidelines for Americans,[2] moderate alcohol consumption is defined as up to 1 drink per day for women and up to 2 drinks per day for men. Know that even if you drink within these limits, you could have problems with alcohol if you drink too quickly, have health conditions, or take medications. If you are pregnant or may become pregnant, you should not drink alcohol.

Heavy or at-risk drinking for women is the consumption of more than 3 drinks on any day or more than 7 per week, and for men it is more than 4 drinks on any day or more than 14 per week. This pattern of drinking too much, too often, is associated with an increased risk for alcohol use disorders. Binge drinking for women is having 4 or more drinks within 2 hours; for men, it is 5 or more drinks within 2 hours. This dangerous pattern of drinking typically results in a BAC of .08% for the average adult and increases the risk of immediate adverse consequences.

What Should I Do If I Suspect Someone Has Alcohol Poisoning?

- » Know the danger signals
- » Do not wait for someone to have all the symptoms
- » Be aware that a person who has passed out may die
- » If you suspect an alcohol overdose, call 911 for help

What Can Happen to Someone With Alcohol Poisoning That Goes Untreated?

- » Choking on his or her own vomit
- » Breathing that slows, becomes irregular, or stops
- » Heart that beats irregularly or stops
- » Hypothermia (low body temperature)
- » Hypoglycemia (too little blood sugar), which leads to seizures
- » Untreated severe dehydration from vomiting, which can cause seizures, permanent brain damage, and death

For more information, please visit: www.niaaa.nih.gov.

[1] Chen, C.M.; Yi, H-y.; and Faden, V.B. *Surveillance Report No. 101: Trends in Underage Drinking in the United States, 1991–2013.* Rockville, MD: National Institute on Alcohol Abuse and Alcoholism, 2015. Available at: http://pubs.niaaa.nih.gov/publications/surveillance101/Underage13.htm.

[2] U.S. Department of Agriculture (USDA) and U.S. Department of Health and Human Services (HHS). *Dietary Guidelines for Americans, 2010.* 7th Edition. Washington, DC: USDA and HHS, 2010, p. 31. Available at: http://www.health.gov/dietaryguidelines/dga2010/DietaryGuidelines2010.pdf.

Figure 10

NEW YORK STATE DEPARTMENT OF HEALTH

Authorization for Release of Health Information (Including Alcohol/Drug Treatment and Mental Health Information) and Confidential HIV/AIDS-related Information

Patient Name	Date of Birth	Patient Identification Number
Patient Address		

I, or my authorized representative, request that health information regarding my care and treatment be released as set forth on this form. I understand that:

1. This authorization may include disclosure of information relating to ALCOHOL and DRUG TREATMENT, MENTAL HEALTH TREATMENT, and CONFIDENTIAL HIV/AIDS-RELATED INFORMATION only if I place my initials on the appropriate line in item 8. In the event the health information described below includes any of these types of information, and I initial the line on the box in Item 8, I specifically authorize release of such information to the person(s) indicated in Item 6.
2. With some exceptions, health information once disclosed may be re-disclosed by the recipient. If I am authorizing the release of HIV/AIDS-related, alcohol or drug treatment, or mental health treatment information, the recipient is prohibited from re-disclosing such information or using the disclosed information for any other purpose without my authorization unless permitted to do so under federal or state law. If I experience discrimination because of the release or disclosure of HIV/AIDS-related information, I may contact the New York State Division of Human Rights at 1-888-392-3644. This agency is responsible for protecting my rights.
3. I have the right to revoke this authorization at any time by writing to the provider listed below in Item 5. I understand that I may revoke this authorization except to the extent that action has already been taken based on this authorization.
4. Signing this authorization is voluntary. I understand that generally my treatment, payment, enrollment in a health plan, or eligibility for benefits will not be conditional upon my authorization of this disclosure. However, I do understand that I may be denied treatment in some circumstances if I do not sign this consent.

5. Name and Address of Provider or Entity to Release this Information:

6. Name and Address of Person(s) to Whom this Information Will Be Disclosed:

7. Purpose for Release of Information:

8. Unless previously revoked by me, the specific information below may be disclosed from: ____________ (INSERT START DATE) until ____________ (INSERT EXPIRATION DATE OR EVENT)

☐ All health information (written and oral), except:

For the following to be included, indicate the specific information to be disclosed and initial below.	Information to be Disclosed	Initials
☐ Records from alcohol/drug treatment programs		
☐ Clinical records from mental health programs*		
☐ HIV/AIDS-related Information		

9. If not the patient, name of person signing form:	10. Authority to sign on behalf of patient:

All items on this form have been completed, my questions about this form have been answered and I have been provided a copy of the form.

SIGNATURE OF PATIENT OR REPRESENTATIVE AUTHORIZED BY LAW — DATE

Witness Statement/Signature: I have witnessed the execution of this authorization and state that a copy of the signed authorization was provided to the patient and/or the patient's authorized representative.

STAFF PERSON'S NAME AND TITLE — SIGNATURE — DATE

This form may be used in place of DOH-2557 and has been approved by the NYS Office of Mental Health and NYS Office of Alcoholism and Substance Abuse Services to permit release of health information. However, this form does not require health care providers to release health information. Alcohol/drug treatment-related information or confidential HIV-related information released through this form must be accompanied by the required statements regarding prohibition of re-disclosure.

*Note: Information from mental health clinical records may be released pursuant to this authorization to the parties identified herein who have a demonstrable need for the information, provided that the disclosure will not reasonably be expected to be detrimental to the patient or another person.

DOH-5032 (6/11)

Acknowledgements

I would like to thank Ruth Bollo for her inspiration and guidance. You have taught me to see everyday as an opportunity to live life to its fullest. Your friendship has been invaluable.

To Anne Akers, my acquisition editor, you have guided me each step of the way, and this book would not have been possible without your experience and encouragement.

To Allen and Peter Adamson - your expertise and critical input have helped me make this book something I can truly be proud of.

About The Author:

Dr. Jacqueline Jones

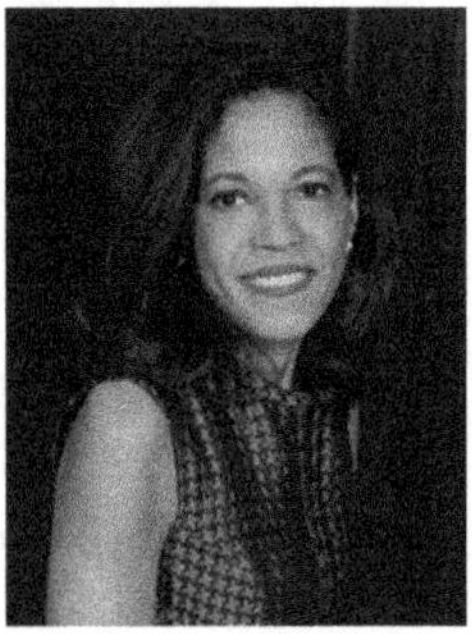

As the mother of two grown children Dr. Jones has navigated the medical system with her own children. Her expertise as a physician and surgeon with over 25 years experience make her uniquely qualified to give parents meaningful advice. Dr. Jones trained as a physician at Cornell Medical College as well as completing her surgical training at University of Pennsylvania and Harvard Medical School. She is listed as one of America's Top doctors and is a Clinical Associate Professor at Weill Cornell Medical College. She is a fellow of the American Academy of Pediatrics and American College of Surgeons.

- Best Doctors in America
- Castle and Connolly Top Doctors
- Top 100 Black Doctors in America
- Talk of the Town Award
- Compassionate Physician Award
- Yelp Patient Satisfaction Award
- Who's Who in America
- Fellow of the American Academy of Pediatrics
- Fellow of the American College of Surgeons
- American Medical Association
- American Society of Pediatric Otolaryngology
- American Academy of Otolaryngology/ Head and Neck Surgery

Bibliography

1. Turck D, Vidailhet M, Bocquet A, et al. Breastfeeding: health benefits for child and mother. *Arch Pediatr.* 2013;20 (suppl):29-48.
2. Morris BJ, Gray R, Castellsague XR, et al. The Strong Protective Effect of Circumcision against Cancer of the Penis. *Advances in Urology*. 2011; (10): 1-21.
3. Kain Z, Mayes L, Caldwell-Andrews A, et al. Preoperative Anxiety, Postoperative Pain, and Behavioral Recovery in Young Children Undergoing Surgery. *Pediatrics*. 2006;118 (2):651-658.
4. Rabbitts JA, Fisher E, Rosenbloom BN, et al. Prevalence and Predictors of Chronic Postsurgical Pain in Children: A Systematic Review and Meta-Analysis. *The Journal of Pain*. 2017;18 (6):605-614.
5. Sun LS, Li G, Miller TL, et al. Association Between a Single General Anesthesia Exposure Before Age 36 Months and Neurocognitive Outcomes in Later Childhood. *JAMA*. 2016; 315(21): 2312-2320.
6. Compas G, Jaser S, Dunn M, et al. Coping with Chronic Illness in Childhood and Adolescence. *Annual Review of Clinical Psychology*. 2012;8:455-480.
7. Revel D. *Pediatric Dental Health*. Dental Resource.org. http://dental-resource.org/topics10.htm. Updated 2006. Accessed Nov. 2017.
8. Seow WK. Enamel hypoplasia in the primary dentition: a review. *ASDC J Dent Child.*1991; 58 (6): 441-52.
9. Tham R, Bowatte G, et al. Breastfeeding and the risk of dental caries: a systematic review and meta-analysis. *Acta Paediiatr*. 2015;104(468):62-84.
10. Peres K, Nascimento G, Peres M, et al. Impact of Prolonged Breastfeeding on Dental Caries: A Population-Based Birth Cohort Study. *Pediatrics*. 2017;140 (1):2016-2943.
11. Li Y, Caufield P. The Fidelity of Initial Acquisition of Mutans

Streptococci by Infants from Their Mothers. *Journal of Dental Research.* 1995;74(2):681-685.

12. Camoin A, Tardieu C, Blanchet I, et al. Sleep bruxism in children. *Archives of Pediatrics.* 2017;24:659-666.
13. Vandenplas Y, Brueton M, Dupont C, et al. Guidelines for the diagnosis and management of cow's mild protein allergy in infants. *Arch Dis Child.* 2007; 92 (10): 902-908.
14. Stice E, Marti CN, Shaw H, et al. An 8-year longitudinal study of the natural history of threshold, subthreshold, and partial eating disorders from a community sample of adolescents. *J Abnorm Psychol.* 2010;118(3):587-597.
15. Amianto F, Ottone L, Abbate Daga G, et al Binge-eating disorder diagnosis and treatment: a recap in front of DSM-5. *BMC Psychiatry.* 2015;15:70. doi: 10.1186/s12888-015-0445-6.Accessed Nov 2017.
16. Birch LL, Fisher JO. Development of eating behaviors among children and adolescents. *Pediatrics.*1998;101(3 Pt 2):539-549.
17. Stice E, Bohon C. Eating Disorders. In Beauchaine T, Linshaw S, eds *Child and Adolescent Psychopathology*, 2nd Edition. Hoboken,NJ: Wiley;2016: 818-838.
18. Smink FE, Van Hoeken D, Hoek HW. Epidemiology of eating disorders: Incidence, prevalence and mortality rates. *Current Psychiatry Reports.* 2012;14(4):406-414.
19. Stice E, Agras W, Hammer LD. Risk factors for the emergence of childhood eating disturbances: a five-year prospective study. *Int J Eat Disord.*1999;25(4):375-87.
20. Marks A, Rothbart B. *Healthy Teens, Body and Soul: A Parent's Complete Guide.* New York, NY: Simon and Schuster; 2003.
21. Livingston G. Stay-at-home moms and dads account for one-in-five U.S. parents. Fact Tank. Pew Research Center. http://www.pewresearch.org/fact-tank/2018/09/24/stay-at-home-moms-and-dads-account-for-about-one-in-five-u-s-parents/. Published Sept. 24, 2018. Accessed Dec. 2018.
22. Statistics on stay-at-home dads. National At-Home Dad Network. http://athomedad.org/media-resources/statistics. Accessed Dec. 2018.
23. Parker K, Livingston G. 7 facts about stay-at-home dads. Fact Tank. Pew Research Center. http://www.pewresearch.org/fact-tank/2018/06/13/fathers-day-facts/. Published Jun. 2018. Accessed Dec. 2018.

24. Mendes E, Saad L, McGeeney K. Stay-at-home moms report more depression, sadness, anger: but low-income stay-at-home moms struggle the most. Well-Being. Gallup. news.gallup.com/poll/154685/stay-home-moms-report-depression-sadness-anger.aspx. Published May 18, 2012. Accessed Dec. 2018.
25. Pahr K. Understanding and combating stay at home mom depression. Paste Magazine. www.pastemagazine.com/articles/2017/01/understand-ing-and-combating-stay-at-home-mom-depre.html. Published Jan. 13, 2017. Accessed Dec. 2018.
26. Fall Semester—A Time for Parents to Discuss the Risks of College Drinking. National Institute on Alcohol Abuse and Alcoholism. https://pubs.niaaa.nih.gov/publications/CollegeFactSheet/back_to_ collegeFact.htm. Published Oct. 2016. Accessed Nov. 2017.
27. Wechsler H, Dowdall GW, Maenner G, et al. Changes in Binge Drinking and Related Problems Among American College Students Between 1993 and 1997. Results of the Harvard School of Public Health College Alcohol Study. J Am Coll Health. 1998;47(2):68. doi:10.1080/07448489809595621. Published Aug. 2018. Accessed Dec. 2018.
28. College Drinking. National Institute on Alcohol Abuse and Alcoholism. https://www.niaaa.nih.gov/alcohol-health/special-pop-ulations-co-occurring-disorders/college-drinking. Published Dec. 2015. Accessed Oct. 2017.
29. Park A, Sher KJ, Krull JL. Risky drinking in college changes as fraternity/sorority affiliation changes: A person-environment perspective. *Psychol Addict Behav*. 2008.22(2): 219-229. doi:10.1037/0893-164x.22.2.219. Published Jun. 2008. Accessed Dec. 2017.
30. 2015 Annual Report. Center for Collegiate Mental Health.Publica-tion No. STA 15-108). doi:10.15868/socialsector.25635. Published 2015. Accessed Nov. 2017.
31. Gallese V, Fadiga L, Fogassi L, et al. Action recognition in the premotor cortex. *Brain*.1996;119;(2):593–609.
32. Cattaneo L, Rizzolatti G. The Mirror Neuron System. *Arch Neurol.* 2009;66 (5): 557-560 doi:10.1001/archneurol.2009.41. Accessed Dec. 2017.
33. Brown J. Can Friendships Survive Parenthood? *Parents*. 2017. https://

www.parents.com/parenting/relationships/friendship/can-friendships-survive-parenthood.Accessed Dec. 2017.

34. Bloom L, Bloom C. *101 things I wish I knew when I got married: simple lessons to make love last.* Novato, CA: New World Library, 2004.

Figures

Fig. 1: Pasquini S. Physician Assistant vs. Nurse Practitioner vs. Medical Doctor. *The Physician Assistant Life*. Nov. 2017;26. https://www.thepalife.com/physician-assistant-vs-nurse-practitioner-vs-medical-doctor. Accessed Nov. 2017.

Fig. 2: Keeping your mouth healthy during pregnancy. *J Am Dent Assoc* .2013,144(11):1314. doi:10.14219/jada.archive.2013.0061. Accessed Oct. 2017.

Fig. 3: Eruption chart of Primary and Secondary Teeth. American Dental Association. Mouth Healthy. 2017. http://www.mouthhealthy.org/en/az-topics/e/eruption-charts. Accessed Nov. 2017. © American Dental Association. Used with permission.

Fig. 4: Authorization for Release of Medical Information to Parents or Guardians

Fig. 5: Parents' Guide to the Family Educational Rights and Privacy Act: Rights Regarding Children's Education Records. 2007.U.S. Department of Education. https://www2.ed.gov/policy/gen/guid/fpco/brochures/parents.html. Accessed December 2017.
Ferpa form: U.S. Department of Education "Model Form for Disclosure to Parents of Dependent Students and Consent Form for Disclosure to Parents. 2007. http://www2.edu.gov/modelform-2html.Accessed Dec .2017.